AF598102

Lithotripsy - Novel Technologies, Innovations and Contemporary Applications

Edited by Mohammad Hammad Ather, Athanasios Papatsoris and Srinath K. Chandrasekara

Published in London, United Kingdom

Lithotripsy - Novel Technologies, Innovations and Contemporary Applications
http://dx.doi.org/10.5772/intechopen.111145
Edited by Mohammad Hammad Ather, Athanasios Papatsoris and Srinath K. Chandrasekara

Contributors
Syed Muhammad Nazim, Liaqat Ali, Faiza Hayat, Nasir Orakzai, Syeda Asiya Hassan, Danya Ali, Jian James Zhang, Victor Enrique Corona-Montes, Vanessa Júarez-Cataneo, Juan Eduardo Sánchez-Núñez, Charalambos Kypraios, Ioannis Xoxakos, Ntiela Ntonta, Ioannis Efthimiou, Erhan Erdogan, Kemal Sarica

First published in London, United Kingdom, 2024 by IntechOpen
IntechOpen is the global imprint of INTECHOPEN LIMITED, registered in England and Wales, registration number: 11086078, 5 Princes Gate Court, London, SW7 2QJ, United Kingdom

British Library Cataloguing-in-Publication Data
A catalogue record for this book is available from the British Library

Additional hard and PDF copies can be obtained from orders@intechopen.com

Lithotripsy - Novel Technologies, Innovations and Contemporary Applications
Edited by Mohammad Hammad Ather, Athanasios Papatsoris and Srinath K. Chandrasekara
p. cm.
Print ISBN 978-0-85466-101-5
Online ISBN 978-0-85466-100-8
eBook (PDF) ISBN 978-0-85466-102-2

For EU product safety concerns:
IN TECH d.o.o., Prolaz Marije Krucifikse Kozulić 3, 51000 Rijeka, Croatia,
info@intechopen.com or visit our website at intechopen.com.

Meet the editors

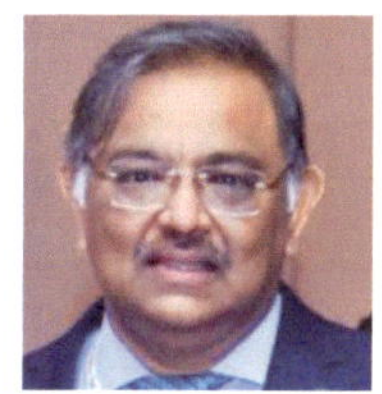

Dr. Mohammad Hammad Ather is a Professor of Urology at Aga Khan University, Pakistan. He is an editorial board member of many international urological journals and author of more than 130 articles in international peer-reviewed journals. He has also written ten book chapters and edited three books. He is an adviser and reviewer for more than two dozen international urological journals and for dissertations and theses at various universities nationally and internationally. He is the founding director of the Conceptual Basis of Urology Course for the Pakistan Association of Urological Surgeons. His research interests include uro oncology, urolithiasis, and training in urology. His main clinical interests include endourology and uro oncology in bladder cancer.

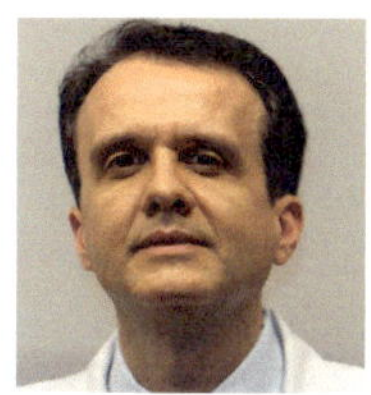

Dr. Athanasios (Thanos) Papatsoris is a Full Professor of Urology at Athens University, Greece. He is also a Visiting Full Professor of Urology at Lebanese University; an adjunct professor at Guangzhou Medical University, China, and the Icahn School of Medicine, USA; a visiting professor at University Basrah Medical College, Iraq, and Rwanda University; an invited professor at the University of Medicine Tirana, Albania; and Scientific Collaborator at the European University of Cyprus. He completed a two-year fellowship in endourology and laparoscopy in London and France. He is a board member of EMA, IAU, HUA, IMBE, and HGUCG. He is an associate board member of ESOU, EULIS, ESUT, ESAU, SEGUR, and U-Merge. He has more than 250 publications to his credit. Dr. Papatsoris is the recipient of the "Arthur Smith" award and chairman of the biannual ESD Congress.

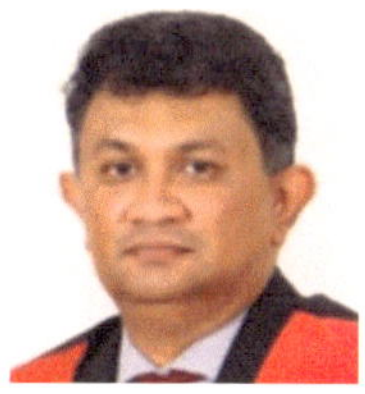

Srinath K. Chandrasekera is a Professor of Surgery and Consultant Urologist in the Department of Surgery, Faculty of the Medical Sciences, University of Sri Jayewardenepura, Sri Lanka. He is a national trainer in postgraduate urological surgery. Previously, Dr. Chandrasekera was the secretary of the College of Surgeons, Sri Lanka Association of Urological Surgeons, and the secretary of the specialist training board of urological surgery. He obtained his training through PGIM and Kings College Hospital London.

Contents

Preface

This book contains exciting new data that will enrich the existing knowledge of those treating stone patients.

Lithotripsy can be performed with various innovative techniques. Scopes, disposables, and fragmentation devices and sources have all seen tremendous progress in the last three decades. The scopes have become finer, fiberoptics technology has considerably advanced, and chip-on-the-tip technology (digital) scopes have tremendously improved the imaging of stones. The use of disposable scopes with fine and highly flexible baskets has improved "stone catching and retrieval." However, one of the most significant improvements which have significantly impacted the safety of endourology in the management of stones is the fragmentation of energy sources. Electrohydraulic and ultrasound were initially replaced by pneumatic devices, and now we have highly efficient, safe, and fine laser fibers for the management of urolithiasis.

This book discusses advancements in extracorporeal shock wave lithotripsy (SWL), such as high-frequency or "burst" SWL. It also presents an in-depth evaluation of standard and novel laser systems, such as thulium lasers, discussing their pros and cons and comparing them to standard holmium lasers. This is of great clinical value for young colleagues who practice laser lithotripsy in semi-rigid and/or flexible (reusable or disposable) ureteroscopic operations. Moreover, for stone surgeons that perform standard or mini percutaneous nephrolithotomy (PCNL), solely or in combination with ureteroscopy (endoscopic combined intrarenal surgery; ECIRS), the book presents useful information regarding the new ultrasound and pneumatic lithotripters. Finally, special attention is given to treating pediatric patients with stone disease in terms of modern technologies, innovations, and contemporary applications of lithotripsy. As such, this book is a useful resource for stone surgeons.

Hammad Ather
Department of Surgery,
Aga Khan University
Karachi, Pakistan

Athanasios Papatsoris
Department of Urology,
Athens University
Athens, Greece

Srinath Chandrasekera
Department of Surgery,
University of Sri Jayewardenepura,
Colombo, Sri Lanka

Section 1

Extracorporeal Shock Wave Lithotripsy

Chapter 1

Advancements in Shock Wave Lithotripsy: Pushing Boundaries with Innovative Technology and Techniques

Syed Muhammad Nazim

Abstract

This chapter explores the significant progress made in shock wave lithotripsy (SWL) for the treatment of urinary tract stones. SWL, a non-invasive treatment modality that uses shock waves to break up stones, is widely employed for urolithiasis treatment. A comprehensive overview of the development of SWL, driven by innovative technology and refined techniques is highlighted. These advancements encompass improvements in lithotripter design, imaging methods, and treatment planning. Notable topics include modifications in shock wave generation, focusing and localization techniques, as well as the clinical application of high-frequency shock waves or 'burst-SWL' that may revolutionize treatment outcomes. The impact of these techniques on treatment effectiveness, stone clearance, safety, potential complications, and patient comfort are also discussed. Furthermore, it delves into the challenges and limitations associated with SWL, such as the importance of tailoring treatment protocols to individual patient needs and considering cost-effectiveness in the era of advanced endo-urology.

Keywords: shockwave lithotripsy, advancement, innovation, technology, design, imaging, outcome

1. Introduction and historical background

The phenomenon of sound waves being focused has been recognized since ancient times. Greeks utilized this knowledge to construct vaults enabling them to overhear on conversations of imprisoned rivals [1]. For decades, high-energy shockwaves have been acknowledged, encompassing blast effects linked to explosions and the sonic boom resulting in window breakage when aircraft surpass the speed of sound [1].

Established by the German Ministry of Defense in 1969, engineers at Dornier Medical Systems commenced investigating shockwave effects on tissues. Not only could they generate shockwaves, but they also discovered that these waves, when generated in water, could traverse living tissues without causing apparent harm; however, brittle materials in their path tended to fracture. This discovery laid the groundwork for the medical application of shockwaves [2]. After achieving the capability to produce low-energy shockwaves in a reproducible and predictable manner, Dornier lithotripter progressed through several prototypes and eventually in February 1980 resulted in first treatment of a human by shock wave lithotripsy (SWL). This was followed by subsequent production and distribution of Dornier HM3 ™ lithotripter in 1983 and approval by the US Food and Drug Administration (FDA) in 1984 [2]. Since then, this approach has emerged as the primary treatment for the majority of urolithiasis patients due to its minimally invasive nature compared to traditional treatments.

The competitive landscape in stone management has shifted. With advancements in endo-urological procedures and more predictable outcomes using alternative methods such as flexible ureteroscopy (f-URS) and percutaneous nephrolithotomy (PCNL), there's a trend moving away from SWL, as technical advancements in SWL have not kept pace with endo-urological progress [1]. This shift is also influenced by diverse practice patterns, evolving indications, facility accessibility, improved instruments in urological arsenal, financial considerations, and urologist preferences [1, 3]. While SWL remains a valuable option for certain patients, its limitation has become increasingly evident. Given these challenges, it is imperative to enhance SWL to maintain its relevance and competitiveness. These include not only continued technological advancements in machine itself but also research into refining patient selection criteria and combining SWL with adjuvant therapies. We explored English language literature pertinent to the topic of advancement in SWL, utilizing electronic databases such as PubMed, ScienceDirect, Google Scholar, and Embase for the compilation of this book chapter.

2. Fundamentals of shock wave lithotripsy (SWL) physics

Shockwaves (SW) are specialized sound waves characterized by a sharp positive pressure peak followed by a trailing negative wave. These waves are generated extracorporeally and passed through the body to fragment stones. SWL operates based on the principles of acoustic energy propagation, focusing, and interaction with stones to induce fragmentation. These waves travel unimpeded through substances with similar acoustic impedance. Upon encountering a boundary between substances with different acoustic impedance, such as water and stone, new stress waves are generated and propagated into the stone [3] This leads to stone fragmentation through compression and tensile forces, erosion, shearing, cavitation, and dynamic fatigue.

In cavitation, when SW energy is applied at a focal point, it results in the formation of water vapor bubbles that explosively collapse, generating microjets that erode and fragment the stone (**Figure 1**).

3. Types of lithotripters

Three types of shockwave generators are available: electrohydraulic (EH), electromagnetic (EM), and piezoelectric (PE) (**Figure 2**). Depending upon the type, various focusing systems are employed to direct this acoustic energy toward a geometric position typically housing the target i.e. stone of interest. Thus shockwaves generated at the first focal point 'F1' are converged at the second focal point 'F2'. The target area (blast path) is a three-dimensional region at 'F2' where shockwaves are concentrated, leading to stone fragmentation [4].

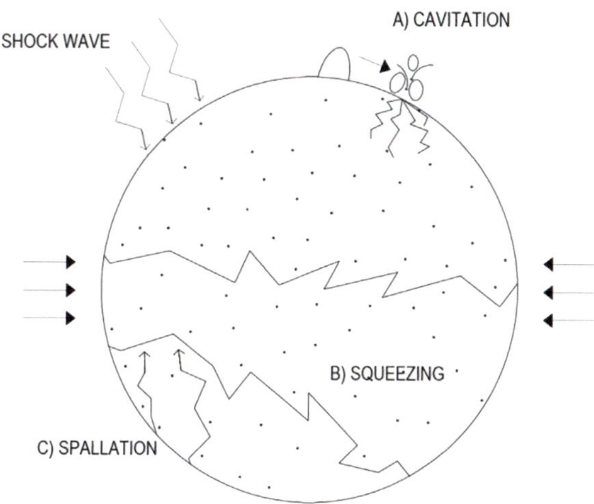

Figure 1.
Shock wave fragmentation effect on stone.

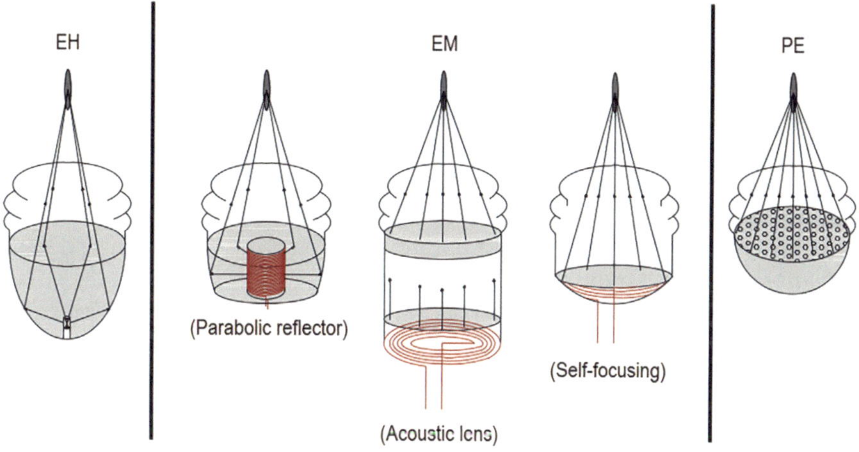

Figure 2.
Different types of shockwave lithotripters. Electrohydraulic (EH), electromagnetic (EM) and Peizoelectric (PE).

3.1 Electrohydraulic (EH) lithotripters

EH lithotripters employ electric discharges to generate shockwaves for stone fragmentation. The original Dornier HM3™ lithotripter utilized this technology, generating shockwaves through an electric spark gap located within a water bath filled with degassed, deionized water. The spark discharge between two electrodes creates a vaporization bubble that expands and collapses, generating a pressure wave [4]. This wave is directed from an ellipsoidal reflector toward the calculus at focal point 'F2'. Although it offered efficient stone fragmentation and versatility, it has relatively shorter-lasting electrodes with the requirement for general anesthesia. Electroconductive (EC) generators are a variant of EH technology, utilizing highly conductive solutions (carbon-based materials, such as graphite or carbon fiber composites) to reduce spark variation and enhancing shockwave delivery efficiency [5].

3.2 Electromagnetic (EM) lithotripters

These devices employ a high-voltage electromagnetic coil to create a magnetic field, inducing vibration in an adjacent metallic membrane, located within a cylindrical 'shock tube' [3, 6]. The resulting shockwave passes through water and is focused at focal point 'F2' using an acoustic lens (Dornier™ and Siemens™) or a parabolic reflector (Storz™). These devices offer reliable shockwave delivery and flexibility in energy adjustments, with the advantage of reduced anesthesia needs and precise targeting [4].

3.3 Piezoelectric (PE) lithotripters

Piezoelectric lithotripters employ multiple piezo-ceramic elements to generate shockwaves. Mounted on a hemispherical dish, these elements expand when excited by high-frequency, high-voltage pulses, generating ultrasonic waves which converge toward the geometric focus of hemispherical carrier, forming a high-energy shockwave [7]. PE lithotripters have a wide area of shockwave entry at the skin surface, causing minimal discomfort, but possess a narrow focal point with limited energy at 'F2', resulting in poorer comminution efficiency. The newer Wolf Piezolith 3000 ™ employs a double layer of piezo-ceramic elements to address this limitation [3].

3.4 Comparison between different types of lithotripters

Each type of shockwave lithotripter comes with its own set of potential advantages and disadvantages. Electrohydraulic (EH) lithotripters, for instance, offer the advantage of producing high-energy shockwaves, making them highly effective for breaking up harder stones. However, they tend to be bulky and require frequent maintenance. Electromagnetic (EM) generators, on the other hand, demand less maintenance, rendering them suitable for outpatient settings. However, they may lack the energy required for larger or denser stones. Piezoelectric (PE) lithotripters provide precise control over shockwave parameters, enhancing safety, but they are generally less powerful. Most comparative studies have focused on EH and EM lithotripters, assessing their efficacy and safety. In a meta-analysis of published reports for the treatment of renal stones <2 cm, EM lithotripters demonstrated a stone-free rate of 70.1%, a re-treatment rate of 46.26%, and a complication rate of 19.7%. In comparison, EH lithotripters exhibited rates of 51.22, 41.6, and 18.8%, respectively. PE lithotripters, while less successful in terms of stone clearance and associated with a higher re-treatment rate, were found to be safer in terms of complications [6].

4. Advancement in lithotripter design

Advancements in SWL technology have been made to enhance its effectiveness and safety, encompassing shockwave generation, focusing, patient coupling, stone localization (imaging), improving efficiency in stone fragmentation and clearance, and strategies to minimize collateral tissue damage.

The original Dornier HM3 ™ lithotripter featured a cumbersome gantry and water bath. Contemporary lithotripters have evolved into smaller, compact, and portable devices [4]. This has enabled performing lithotripsy in diverse positions such as supine, prone, lateral, inclined, or declined leading to increased patient comfort.

Lateral panels incorporate monitors for ultrasound imaging, ECG, and respiratory triggering. Newer lithotripters now use a modular design, separating the fluoroscopy unit from the lithotripter, optimizing storage space, and allowing the fluoroscopy unit's versatility for other procedures [4].

With the evolution, the operators possess the ability to control various device parameters that influence treatment outcomes, including the lithotripter's acoustic output, focal volume, coupling to the patient, SW administration parameters (rate, voltage, sequence & ramping), stone localization and anesthetic technique(s).

5. Advancement in stone localization; innovative imaging techniques for enhanced stone targeting

Accurate stone localization holds paramount importance for the success of SWL procedures and can be achieved through fluoroscopy & ultrasonography.

5.1 Fluoroscopy

Fluoroscopy provides operator with a familiar modality, particularly advantageous for effective ureteral stone localization. However, drawbacks of fluoroscopy include exposure to ionizing radiation for patients and operators, its incapability to locate radiolucent stones and space requirements. Advancements in fluoroscopy technology like digital fluoroscopy and low-dose fluoroscopy offer improved image quality with minimized exposure [8]. Additional technological advances include use of collimators, reducing radiation fields, employing dose level settings, and utilizing pulse fluoroscopy for radiation exposure management by adhering to ALARA (As Low As Reasonably Achievable) principle. The latest lithotripter generations mitigate radiation exposure through automated fluoroscopic localization with improved resolution [8].

5.2 Ultrasound

Ultrasonic stone localization offers real-time monitoring without radiation exposure and can effectively identify radiolucent stones and stone fragments as small as 2–3 mm. Recent ultrasonography advancements, such as high-frequency transducers and improved image resolution, bolster stone localization accuracy. Ultrasound's multi-plane visualization aids in precise targeting and monitoring during shockwave application. Additionally, doppler ultrasound can assess renal blood flow and potential complications such as bleeding and renal hematoma formation. Spectral doppler signal can also provide real-time feedback (hit and miss) information during therapy (Dornier Gemini™) [9].

European Association of Urology (EAU) guidelines suggest both ultrasound and fluoroscopy as valid alternatives to monitor SWL progress [10]. Many new lithotripters combine fluoroscopy and real-time monitoring through ultrasound to reduce imaging radiation exposure. This dual-modality imaging offers enhanced stone localization and treatment precision [8].

As the targeted stones may move out of shockwave focus due to stone or patient movement, shock wave focus/target should be reconfirmed at regular intervals, and continuous ultrasound monitoring or periodic checks every 300 to 500 shocks are recommended [10].

5.3 Virtual tracking system

Stone movement in and out of the focal zone, often due to respiratory and patient movements, impacts fragmentation efficacy. Due to factors such as respiratory rate and excursion length and lower focal width of the SWL machine, the stone may be outside the focal zone during over 50% of SWL sessions [1]. This leads to missed targets and inadvertent renal tissue impacts.

The emergence of virtual tracking systems (VTS) signifies a novel imaging modality that enhances the accuracy and effectiveness of SWL for urolithiasis. Through real-time imaging, tracking technology, and predictive algorithms, VTS achieves precise stone localization and enables targeted shockwave delivery. These systems utilize advanced fluoroscopy and ultrasound-based imaging techniques with sophisticated transducers to track stone position and movement during SWL [1]. Advanced image processing algorithms and built-in systems in piezo-electric lithotripters identify the stone, continuously track its trajectory, and steer the shock waves onto the target [11].

Visio-track (VT) ™ locking system utilizes a handheld probe with infra-red stereo vision to triangulate stone location, adjusting the focal points for enhanced accuracy compensating for respiratory motion, leading to better stone-free rates (79.5% vs. 54.5%, $p = 0.001$) compared to fluoroscopy [12]. Storz Medical™ has 2 tracking options available, acoustic and optical, with the latter proving superior results. EDAP/TMS Sonolith i-sys™ also employs ultrasound imaging complemented by optical tracking for stone localization [12].

Own et al. [13] introduced a real-time tracking and targeting system where short ultrasonic pulses are delivered to the lithotripter's focal point, detecting scattered pulses by a receiver transducer from the stone upon target impact. While these systems show promise, they are still undergoing modifications and have not yet gained widespread clinical adoption.

5.4 Evaluating stone breakage with acoustic feedback

Despite the significant improvement in fluoroscopic and ultrasound imaging for precise stone localization over the years, they remain less reliable in determining treatment endpoints [7]. Experienced urologists recognize signs of stone fragmentation through margin softening, density loss, and particle movement, but these can be challenging to assess.

Acoustic feedback systems have emerged to monitor stone fragmentation [14]. These systems employ a broadband receiver to track shockwaves reflected off the stone, including reverberations from acoustic waves transmitted into the stone. As the stone breaks, smaller fragments generate high-frequency signals. In vitro studies show this system can differentiate fragments varying in size by 1–2 mm thereby minimizing excessive shockwave delivery to renal tissues [14].

Another system by Leighton et al. [15] employs an acoustic sensor to detect emissions from each shock at the lithotripter's focal point. This "listening" device gauges cavitation at the target area, correlating signal quality with stone breakage degree. A computer display indicates if shockwaves hit the stone and whether fragmentation progresses.

5.5 Augmented reality (AR) and virtual reality (VR)

Emerging technologies like augmented reality (AR) and virtual reality (VR) hold potential to transform preoperative planning and intraoperative guidance for shockwave lithotripsy [11]. The integration of AR and robot-assisted ultrasound-guided lithotripsy shows promise for enhancing treatment outcomes and patient care. AR systems overlay virtual information onto real-time ultrasound images, providing augmented visualization and guidance during procedures. Robot-assisted SWL merges robotic precision with real-time ultrasound imaging, enhancing targeting accuracy for shockwave delivery [1].

6. Enhancing treatment strategies and protocols with innovation in technology

To enhance clinical safety and SWL efficiency, extensive research is underway, driven by advancing insights into stone fragmentation mechanisms and tissue injury. The International Alliance of Urolithiasis (IAU) has released comprehensive guidelines for managing urolithiasis, encompassing preoperative evaluation, procedural tips, tricks, and post-procedure follow-up strategies with the aim to provide a clinical framework for urologists engaged in SWL procedures [16].

6.1 Patient and stone-related factors

Despite being non-invasive, SWL encounters limitations and challenges that can influence treatment outcomes. Patient selection significantly influences SWL success rates. Various clinical nomograms aim to identify optimal factors for SWL based on stone-free rates. Predictors encompass clinical parameters like age, sex, body weight, BMI, and CT scan-based factors such as stone location, number, diameter, Hounsfield units (HU), and hydronephrosis presence [16]. One such score is the Triple-D score, utilizing stone diameter, density, and skin-to-stone distance on pre-operative CT scans [17].

Patient-related factors, including obesity (high BMI) and greater skin-to-stone distance, negatively impact SWL success rates [17]. Comparatively, skin-to-stone distance (SSD) outperforms BMI/body weight as a marker of success. Given that most lithotripters possess a 15 cm focal length and adipose tissue attenuates shockwave energy, SSD should not exceed 120 mm [10].

Certain stone compositions, such as brushite, cystine, and calcium oxalate monohydrate, pose challenges to effective fragmentation and may require higher energy level or alternative treatment options. The stone burden is a significant factor that impacts stone free rate (SFR) after SWL. The upper limit for upper tract stones is 20 mm, while for lower pole renal stones, it is 15 mm. Stones with high density (>1000 HU) exhibit resistance to SWL [18]. Stones in anatomically complex sites such as lower calyx stones (with a long infundibulum, narrow infundibular neck, and an acute infundibulopelvic angle), stones in calyceal diverticulum or malformed kidney pose targeting and fragmentation challenges. Lower pole stones treated with SWL tend to have lower clearance rates compared to other collecting system regions. A meta-analysis involving 2927 patients with lower pole stones indicated a decreased stone-free rate (SFR) for SWL (52.9%) compared to PCNL (90%) [19].

6.2 Optimization of SWL parameters

Research has delved into the impact of various shockwave parameters on stone fragmentation, including shockwave energy, frequency, and focal width.

6.2.1 Energy level

The energy level of SW plays a pivotal role in stone fragmentation. Inadequate energy might result in insufficient fragmentation, while excessive energy can lead to tissue injury. Factors such as stone size, composition, and location dictate the suitable energy level.

6.2.2 SW frequency/rate

Ensuring effective stone fragmentation while minimizing harm is essential in SWL. Kidney damage during a single SWL session is dose-dependent on pulse amplitude and shockwave count. The standardized number of shocks per session remains elusive, with a general upper limit of 4000 shocks, subject to energy level used [7].

Lower shockwave doses and slower shockwave rates are recommended to minimize acute and lasting tissue injury. Appropriate shockwave rate can enhance stone fragmentation and limit tissue damage. Dornier HM3 TM, the first clinically used lithotripter, employed a "gated" shockwave rate synchronized with electrocardiogram (ECG), often around 60 to 80 per minute. Subsequent lithotripters shifted to non-gated fixed rates, typically 100–120 per minute, aiming for shorter treatment times [6].

The exact mechanism influencing rate's impact on SWL efficiency is debated but is different for stone breakage and tissue injury [20]. Cavitation bubbles generated during SWL implode against the stone surface, forming high-speed jets that erode it [2]. At higher rates, subsequent shocks hit existing bubbles, creating less effective bubble clouds that absorb/dissipate energy [20].

Renal tissue damage, including hematoma formation, also ties to cavitation effects. Faster shockwave rates than tissue's relaxation time induces stress accumulation and vessel rupture, intensifying cavitation's impact [2]. Numerical models suggest a shockwave threshold for tissue relaxation around 1 Hz, with rates above 60 SW/min causing tissue deformation and injury [2].

Reducing shockwave delivery to 60 per minute from 120 in a randomized controlled trial elevated stone-free rates from 28 to 60% [3]. A meta-analysis comparing 60 vs. 120 shocks per minute confirmed improved success with 60, along with fewer additional procedures and better cost-effectiveness [21].

6.2.3 Focal length and positioning

Proper positioning and focal length of shockwaves are critical for effective stone fragmentation. Focal length determines the distance between the shockwave source and the stone, and it should be adjusted according to the stone's location within the urinary tract [4]. Precise focusing ensures accurate targeting and concentration of shockwaves on the stones. Aligning stone adjustment with the shockwave's focal point enhances treatment efficiency and reduces the risk of collateral damage.

6.2.4 Enhancing stone fragment expulsion using adjuvant pharmacotherapy

A key challenge in SWL is the clearance of residual fragments, often necessitating secondary treatments. Residual stone fragments can lead to complications like Steinstrasse, regrowth, infections, renal colic, and persistent discomfort. Innovations aimed at expediting fragment passage encompass various instruments [2].

Studies have demonstrated the utility of pharmacological therapies to promote stone passage and enhance the overall effectiveness of SWL. These treatments involve calcium channel blockers, corticosteroids, nonsteroidal anti-inflammatory drugs (NSAIDs), and alpha-blockers [20]. These modalities effectively reduce the time and pain associated with stone expulsion.

Although treatment protocols remain to be standardized, multiple studies and meta-analyses demonstrate that mechanical percussion, forced diuresis, and body inversion (PDI) with external physical vibration 'lithecbolc' (EPVL) are safe and effective methods for assisting the clearance of stone fragments, particularly for lower pole stones [22].

PDI therapy contributes to enhanced stone clearance in three ways: increased urine production for fragment flushing, prone Trendelenburg positioning to exploit gravity, and manual/mechanical flank percussion to dislodge fragments *via* vibration.

6.2.5 Focused ultrasound therapy

Advancements in focused ultrasound technology for residual fragment clearance are yielding promising outcomes. Transcutaneous focused ultrasound therapy probe is used to generate acoustic streaming forces sufficient to displace stone fragments by several centimeters [23]. Equipped with an ultrasound imaging probe, this therapy probe locates and directs fragments for clearance. This also aids the dispersion of fragment clusters to ascertain effective stone breakup [6].

6.2.6 Timing and treatment repetition

The decision to repeat treatment depends on the stone's response to the initial session. No prospective study has been conducted to determine the appropriate time interval for repeated shockwave lithotripsy sessions. For kidney stones, the interval between two shockwave sessions should not be less than 1 to 2 weeks. For ureteral stones, an interval of 1 day may suffice. This is attributed to the fact that renal contusions typically improve within 1 to 2 weeks, and there is no evidence that SWL for ureteral stones leads to renal hematoma formation [4].

6.2.7 Improving acoustic coupling

One of the critical parameters to enhance stone fragmentation while minimizing associated SWL side effects is acoustic coupling. The first-generation lithotripter, Dornier HM3™, employed a 1000 L water bath to couple shockwaves to the patient. Water, with an acoustic impedance closely resembling body tissue, efficiently transmits shockwaves into the body, minimizing energy reflection or absorption at the water-skin interface [3].

Subsequent lithotripter generations introduced water cushions with silicon membranes in dry treatment heads. This design improved portability and convenience for both patients and operators. However, these dry treatment heads necessitate coupling media, like gels or oils, to connect the patient to the device. For instance, the use of a water cushion combined with ultrasonic gel replaced the traditional water bath [1, 4]. An exception among current machines is the Storz SLX™ (Storz Medical Switzerland), which employs a partial water bath for shock head coupling. This lithotripter is especially good for obese patients facing issues with coupling efficiency and accurate stone localization [7].

Conventionally, coupling involves applying gel to the treatment head's cushion and patient's skin contact area [7]. Enhancing coupling quality involves improved gel application and handling techniques [20]. Effective application includes directly applying gel from a jug to the treatment head's center, followed by pressing the cushion onto the patient. Further, spreading the gel is facilitated by increasing cushion water inflation pressure [7].

The media's quality and viscosity significantly impact SWL's effectiveness. Studies have shown that higher-quality water-soluble lubricating gel with lower viscosity exhibited superior stone fragmentation with the need for lesser number of shock waves [20]. Minimizing trapped air bubbles in the coupling media is crucial, as these bubbles substantially reduce shockwave efficiency. De-coupling and re-coupling during patient repositioning can introduce substantial air pockets in the coupling medium. Studies indicate that a mere 2% of coupling area occupied by air bubbles leads to a 20 to 40% reduction in stone fragmentation efficiency [24].

Direct imaging provides immediate feedback, while some lithotripters equipped with in-line ultrasound probes monitor coupling [3]. Devices featuring video cameras have been developed to ensure optimal coupling by detecting air bubbles in the transmission zone. Tailly et al. [25] have introduced a modification to acoustic coupling by incorporating a camera and LED light in the shockwave head of a Dornier Gemini ™. This modification has been effective in improving coupling quality, leading to a 25% reduction in number of applied shockwaves and energy. This approach outperformed blind coupling in a study involving 336 patients who underwent SWL (SFR: 78.2% for renal and 81.7% for ureteral stones vs. 62.9% for renal and 67.9% for ureteral stones) ($p < 0.05$) [25].

6.3 Enhancing safety: monitoring and safety measures

While SWL is generally safe, several enhancements have been devised to minimize discomfort, optimize patient compliance, and ensure favorable outcomes. Real-time monitoring of shockwave delivery, patient vital signs, and treatment response has advanced over time. Similarly, adequate pre-hydration, appropriate shockwave parameter selection, maximal shocks per session, and precise focusing are vital [20].

Shockwave delivery monitoring involves tracking shockwave energy, focal point localization, and coupling efficiency. Focal point localization monitoring ensures precise stone targeting, reducing impact on surrounding tissues. Coupling efficiency monitoring evaluates acoustic coupling quality between the shockwave source and patient skin, optimizing energy transmission [25]. Real-time monitoring of patient vital signs and physiological parameters during SWL aids in detecting adverse events and patient discomfort.

6.4 Patient positioning

During SWL, a stable patient position is crucial as patient and respiratory movements can displace stones from the shockwave focus, impairing disintegration rates. Optimal patient positioning is crucial to minimize shockwave travel distance and mitigate interference from skeletal elements such as transverse processes, ribs, sacroiliac bones, and the pelvis [4].

Accessories like neck rolls, knee rolls, wedges, and armrests can stabilize patients. Modern lithotripters offer under-table and over-table positions, enabling supine treatment for all stone locations [16].

6.5 Anesthesia and sedation techniques

Advancements in anesthesia and sedation techniques have significantly improved patient comfort during SWL procedures. By enhancing patient tolerability through analgesia, overall SWL outcomes can be positively influenced.

The initial clinical lithotripter, Dornier HM3™, required general anesthesia for treatment. Subsequent lithotripter generations enable treatment without anesthesia. Newer designs feature wider apertures that distribute the acoustic field over a broader skin area, thereby reducing skin surface pain [2].

Intravenous sedation, often termed conscious sedation, is a well-suited pain management protocol for most SWL patients. This involves administering sedative medications to induce a state of reduced awareness and anxiety during the procedure thus fostering patient cooperation and tolerance during SWL. Commonly used medications include benzodiazepines (e.g., Midazolam) and opioids (e.g., Fentanyl) to achieve conscious sedation.

A meta-analysis of randomized controlled trials assessing opioids, non-steroidal anti-inflammatory drugs (NSAIDs), and simple analgesia (Paracetamol) showed both NSAIDs and opioids provided safe and effective analgesia, with no significant pain score differences [26].

In cases where conscious sedation is not available or complex cases with prolonged procedures are involved, general anesthesia may be necessary. This approach is favored for infants, young children, and extremely anxious patients [2]. General anesthesia also minimizes stone motion by controlling respiratory rate and volume. Studies comparing general anesthesia and conscious sedation for SWL indicated higher success rates (70–87%) in the general anesthesia group compared to 51–55% in sedation group respectively [26].

6.6 Advancement in focal zone and volume

Acoustic output, amplitude, and spatial energy distribution vary between lithotripters [1]. A narrower focal zone dissipates less energy into the stone, particularly if narrower than the stone. Evidence suggests that a wide focal zone benefits stone disintegration through 'dynamic squeezing' by accommodating stone motion and increasing shockwave-stone contact [1, 3].

To address limitations of contemporary electromagnetic lithotripters (with relatively narrower focal zones), modifications to the acoustic lens can be implemented (**Figure 3**). Creating an annular cut on the outer back surface of the acoustic lens generates a second shockwave from the same pulse, leading to "pulse superimposition" in situ [27]. The second wave overlays the first shockwave from the uncut part in the focal area.

Another enhancement involves an "energy-dependent" focal shift of electromagnetic lithotripters, broadening the focal width by using a smaller lens aperture in the uncut area to reach around 11 mm (49%) at a relevant treatment energy level [3].

6.7 Dual head lithotripters and tandem pulse technology

Ongoing efforts in the field of SWL aim to refine stone fragmentation techniques, specifically enhancing the crucial mechanism of stone breakage - cavitation. Cavitation bubbles play an indispensable role in stone comminution, and an

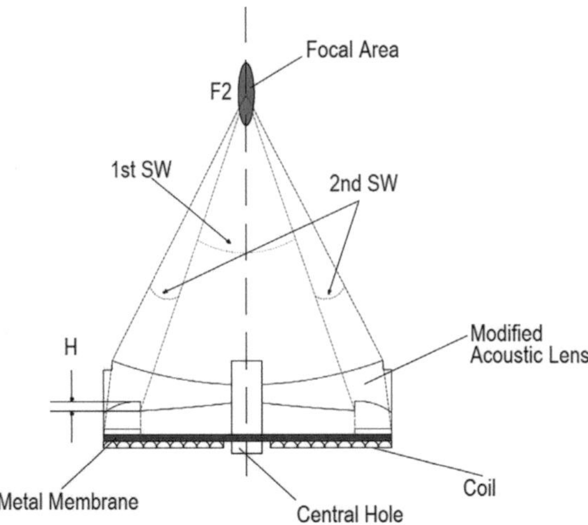

Figure 3.
Modification in acoustic lens of EM lithotripter creating 'pulse superimposition'.

innovative approach involves employing rapid successive shockwaves to forcefully collapse these bubbles against the stone surface [1, 3]. Efforts are directed toward optimizing the efficacy of cavitation bubbles' action on the stone surface. Emerging as an innovative approach to enhance lithotripsy procedures, dual-head lithotripters offer improved efficiency, precision, and effectiveness. The concept of dual lithotripters suggests that energy distribution between two synchronized or alternating sources can improve breakage by manipulating the acoustic field [6].

Research indicates that dual pulses effectively localize and intensify cavitation damage in laboratory settings [2, 6]. These devices incorporate two independent shockwave generation sources positioned on opposite sides of the patient, resulting in overlapping or converging shockwaves that lead to enhanced stone fragmentation, treatment flexibility, and improved treatment efficiency. Synchronous arrival of two pulses at the focal point results in pressure doubling, leading to enhanced bubble growth and greater focal pit depth.

The advantages over traditional single-source lithotripters are manifold. Dual shockwave generation allows for more focused energy delivery, concentrating energy at the targeted stone, thereby boosting fragmentation efficiency. Additionally, by manipulating the intensity and timing of shockwaves from each source, treatment flexibility is enhanced, accommodating different stone sizes and compositions. Simultaneous application of shockwaves from two sources reduces treatment duration, promoting patient comfort while mitigating the risk of complications [1, 7].

Another modification involving a "reflector insert" integrated with the original Dornier HM3™ reflector creates a second shockwave immediately after the first, reducing the negative tensile component and improving stone fragmentation while minimizing vascular and renal parenchymal injury [6]. Storz Modulith SLX F2™ offers a dual focus system to adjust focal size, and an alternative approach involves modifying the pulse duration from an electromagnetic source to increase the focal size [1, 4]. Wolf Piezolith 3000™ employs a double layer of Piezo-ceramic elements to amplify shockwave energy without enlarging the dish [3, 4]. Although dual-head lithotripters are not yet widely adopted, ongoing refinements and further research could pave the way for their broader application in the future.

Tandem pulse lithotripsy is an active area of investigation, showing potential to enhance stone fragmentation while minimizing associated injury. This technology involves a second shockwave succeeding the first along the same acoustic axis to forcefully collapse bubbles against the stone. There are two ways to achieve this. The first involves integrating an auxiliary lithotripter, specifically a Piezo-electric array, to generate a secondary (trailing) shockwave that follows the trajectory of the initial shockwave along the same acoustic axis [3, 6]. The second method entails incorporating a piezo-electric lithotripter with an additional charging and discharge circuit, resulting in the emission of a second pulse - a tandem shockwave [2, 6].

6.8 Optimizing shockwave sequence and power (energy) ramping

The sequence of shockwave delivery relates to timing, numbers, power levels, and power ramping—gradual energy increase during lithotripsy. Power ramping was introduced to acclimatize patients to shockwaves in anesthesia-free lithotripsy.

Power ramping with a short pause not only enhances SWL stone fragmentation but also mitigates renal tissue injury [6, 28]. Low-energy shockwaves during ramping condition stones, improving subsequent high-energy pulse fragmentation. Low-voltage stress waves fragment stones, while high-energy shockwaves lead to greater cavitary activity and further fragmentation [3]. Energy ramping's reno-protective effect is well-supported. Pre-treatment with low-energy shockwaves followed by a pause triggers vasoconstriction, reducing bleeding risk in stiffer vessels, and thus safeguarding against renal injury [20, 28].

In 2016, Skuginna et al. [28] randomized patients with renal stones to stepwise voltage ramping or fixed power. Stepwise ramping reduced renal hematoma rates, with 5.6 vs. 13% in fixed power ($P = 0.008$). Lambert et al. found that ramping protocol SWL led to lower urinary macroglobulin and beta-2 macroglobulin levels, markers of renal injury [29].

Although no standard protocol exists and depends upon operator preference, the preferred approach is to give 100–500 low energy SW and a 3-minute pause before starting the 'clinical dose' of SW therapy [20].

A summary of the technological innovations to enhance lithotripsy effectiveness and safety is presented in **Table 1**.

7. Burst waves and high-frequency shockwaves

The introduction of burst shockwave lithotripsy (BWL) or high-frequency SWL is poised to be a transformative development. Developed at University of Washington, BWL stands as an emerging cutting-edge technology and has the potential to resurge interest in non-invasive treatment approaches for urolithiasis. In an in vitro study, Maxwell et al. [30] demonstrated that this technique enables fine stone fragmentation within a brief timeframe, dependent on stone composition and applied frequency.

In contrast to SWL, where high-amplitude (30–100 MPa) acoustic shocks are applied at slow rate (1–2 Hz) to disintegrate the stone, BWL utilizes low-amplitude (< 12 MPa) bursts of ultrasound delivered at higher frequencies (200 Hz) to repeatedly stress the stones until they ultimately fracture (**Figure 4**). This leads to formation of tiny, uniform-sized fragments separate from the surface of the larger stone body compared to SWL where stones often shatter into larger fragments. These tiny fragments are small enough to pass spontaneously without any additional intervention [31].

Strategy	Summary and examples
Modifications and technological innovations in lithotripter	Attenuating cavitation- induced injury • Direct wave suppression • Modified reflectors insert
	Enhancing Cavitation-induced stone fragmentation • Dual pulse & Tandem Pulse lithotripsy • Dual focus system (Storz Modulith SLX F2) • Double layer of PE elements (Wolf Piezolith 3000)
	Enhancing pre-procedure planning • Augmented reality (AR) and Virtual reality (VR)
	Enhancing stone localization and targeting • Combined modality imaging • Spectral doppler ultrasound (Dornier Gemini™) • Virtual tracking system (Visio-track VT™)
	Advancement in Focal zone and volume • Acoustic lens modification to create 'pulse superimposition'
	Improving acoustic coupling • Partial water bath (Storz SLX™) • Direct imaging with camera and LED (Dornier Gemini™)
	Evaluating stone breakage • Acoustic feedback (Acoustic sensor)- Broadband receiver to track SW reflected off stone
	Enhancing precision and faster stone disintegration • Burst wave lithotripsy (BWL) (Piezoelectric high-frequency soundwave 'packages') • Electrohydraulic high-frequency SW
Modification of treatment strategies and protocols	Proper positioning of patient • Mitigating interference from skeletal elements. • Aligning stone adjustment with SW focal point
	Lowering SW dose and Slowing SW rate • Reducing the dose to 60/min
	Optimizing shockwave sequence • Low voltage pre-treatment ('priming' for first 100–500 SW) • Power ramping (stepwise increase in voltage) • Timing and treatment repetition (1–2 weeks for Kidney stones)

Strategy	Summary and examples
Adjuncts to improve SWL safety and efficacy	Patient selection (Determining SWL success by;) • Stone density (HU) • Skin-to-stone distance (SSD) • Body mass index (BMI) • Renal Anatomy (Lower pole, pelvicalyceal angle, infundibular length)
	Adjuvant pharmacotherapy to improve stone expulsion and reduce pain. • NSAIDS • Alpha-blockers • Calcium channel blockers
	Percussion, Inversion and Diuresis (PID) therapy • Percussion (manual or mechanical) • Inversion (45–70°), and • Diuresis (500 ml of water or 20 mg furosemide with or without 1–2 L of IV fluid)
	Altering the chemical environment surrounding Urine • Urinary alkalinizer

Table 1.
Advancement in shock wave lithotripsy.

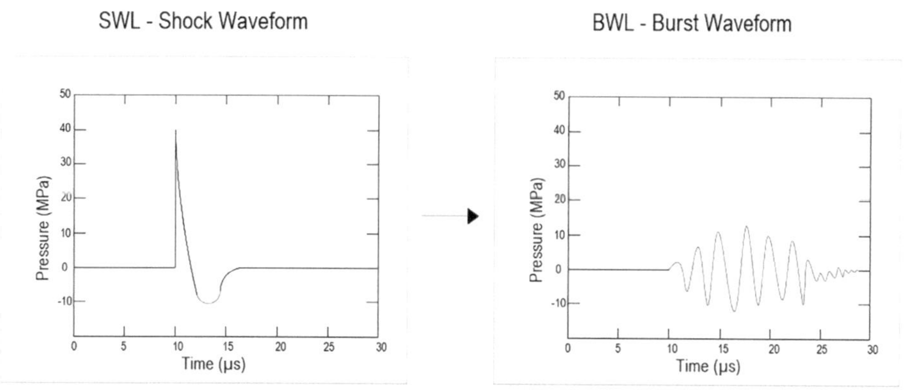

Figure 4.
Pressure waveform of SWL and BWL.

This treatment offers numerous benefits when compared to traditional SWL. This modality can be administered using a handheld probe while the patient is awake in an office setting and limiting radiation exposure. It can target and fragment the stones with remarkable precision and can effectively treat wide range of

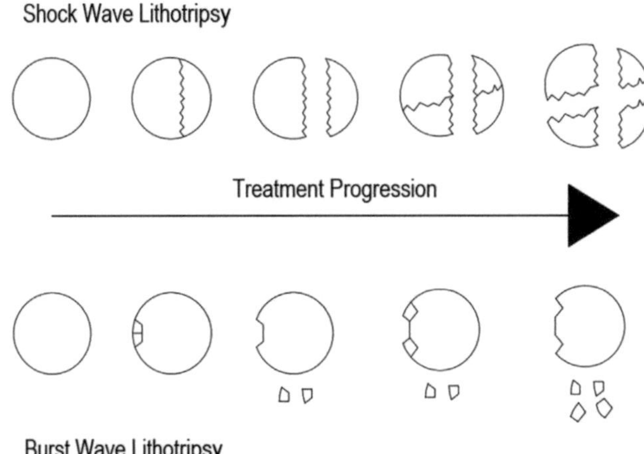

Figure 5.
Stone fragmentation in SWL and BWL.

kidney stone types (**Figure 5**). The reduced formation of cavitation bubbles minimizes tissue injury with lesser pain [31].

Recently, Harper et al. conducted first feasibility study of BWL to evaluate its effectiveness and safety. They used a device Propulse 1™ and handheld, water-filled, combined imaging and therapy transducer, SC-60 ™, that was coupled with gel to the skin allowing simultaneous visualization and comminution or propulsion of kidney stones. They recruited 19 patients with kidney stones <12 mm of varying composition and location. Within just 10 minutes of treatment, most of the stones either completely or partially disintegrated with minimal damage to the surrounding tissues [32].

A synergistic impact on the effectiveness of stone fragmentation is observed when ultrasonic propulsion (UP) is employed alongside BWL. This phenomenon is attributed to the following mechanism: UP can physically expel fragments that are loosely adhered to the stone, as well as reposition the stone and redistribute stress, ultimately resulting in the formation of new stress fractures within the stones [33].

While BWL holds promise and may find its place in the armamentarium of kidney stone treatments, it currently faces challenges related to technical complexity, limited clinical evidence, cost considerations, and competition with established techniques [31]. The lack of standardized protocols and guidelines for BWL could lead to variances in treatment outcomes, impeding its widespread adoption. Further research, refinement of technology, and the accumulation of clinical data may help address these issues and improve the overall success and acceptance of burst wave lithotripsy in the future.

8. Conclusion and future perspectives

SWL remains the non-invasive surgical technique for the treatment of urinary stones. Continuous exploration of SWL physics and the interaction of shockwaves with stones are anticipated to expand the boundaries of SWL and optimize patient outcomes. The future of SWL is expected to be shaped by evolving lithotripter designs, integration of advanced imaging and tracking technologies, refined treatment protocols, and personalized treatment algorithms.

In the era of minimally invasive endo-urology, the meticulous selection of patients assumes a pivotal role in optimizing patient outcomes. As we acknowledge its limitations and embrace technological advancements, SWL can retain its essential role in the diverse landscape of stone management given its non-invasive nature and suitability for outpatient care. The path forward involves adapting and seamlessly integrating SWL into the broader spectrum of stone management techniques, thereby ensuring that patients receive the most suitable and effective treatment tailored to their specific conditions.

Acknowledgements

The author graciously acknowledges contribution of Engineer Syed Muhammad Shakir Fateh, Manager (Protection and Automation) Siemens Pakistan Engineering Company Limited for technical support.

Author details

Syed Muhammad Nazim
The Aga Khan University Hospital, Karachi, Pakistan

*Address all correspondence to: muhammad.nazim@aku.edu

References

[1] Rassweiler J, Rieker P, Rassweiler-Seyfried MC. Extracorporeal shock-wave lithotripsy: Is it still valid in the era of robotic endourology? Can it be more efficient? Current Opinion in Urology. 2020;**30**(2):120-129. DOI: 10.1097/MOU.0000000000000732

[2] Basulto-Martínez M, Klein I, Gutiérrez-Aceves J. The role of extracorporeal shock wave lithotripsy in the future of stone management. Current Opinion in Urology. 2019;**29**(2):96-102. DOI: 10.1097/MOU.0000000000000584

[3] Neisius A, Lipkin ME, Rassweiler JJ, Zhong P, Preminger GM, Knoll T. Shock wave lithotripsy: The new phoenix? World Journal of Urology. 2015;**33**(2):213-221. DOI: 10.1007/s00345-014-1369-3

[4] Lee SM, Collin N, Wiseman H, Philip J. Optimisation of shock wave lithotripsy: A systematic review of technical aspects to improve outcomes. Translational Andrology and Urology. 2019;**8**(Suppl. 4):S389-S397. DOI: 10.21037/tau.2019.06.07

[5] Pemberton RJ, Tolley DA. Comparison of a new-generation electroconductive spark lithotripter and the Dornier Compact Delta for ureteral calculi in a quaternary referral center. Journal of Endourology. 2006;**20**(10):732-736. DOI: 10.1089/end.2006.20.732

[6] Elmansy HE, Lingeman JE. Recent advances in lithotripsy technology and treatment strategies: A systematic review update. International Journal of Surgery. 2016;**36**(Pt. D):676-680. DOI: 10.1016/j.ijsu.2016.11.097

[7] Lingeman JE, McAteer JA, Gnessin E, Evan AP. Shock wave lithotripsy: Advances in technology and technique. Nature Reviews. Urology. 2009;**6**(12):660-670. DOI: 10.1038/nrurol.2009.216

[8] Chang TH, Lin WR, Tsai WK, Chiang PK, Chen M, Tseng JS, et al. Comparison of ultrasound-assisted and pure fluoroscopy-guided extracorporeal shockwave lithotripsy for renal stones. BMC Urology. 2020;**20**(1):183. DOI: 10.1186/s12894-020-00756-6

[9] Bohris C, Bayer T, Lechner C. Hit/miss monitoring of ESWL by spectral Doppler ultrasound. Ultrasound in Medicine & Biology. 2003;**29**(5):705-712. DOI: 10.1016/s0301-5629(02)00773-1

[10] Tzelves L, Türk C, Skolarikos A. European Association of Urology Urolithiasis guidelines: Where are we going? European Urology Focus. 2021;7(1):34-38. DOI: 10.1016/j.euf.2020.09.011

[11] Muller S, Abildsnes H, Ostvik A, Kragset O, Gangås I, Birke H, et al. Can a dinosaur think? Implementation of artificial intelligence in extracorporeal shock wave lithotripsy. European Urology Open Science. 2021;**27**:33-42. DOI: 10.1016/j.euros.2021.02.007

[12] Abid N, Ravier E, Promeyrat X, Codas R, Fehri HF, Crouzet S, et al. Decreased radiation exposure and increased efficacy in extracorporeal lithotripsy using a new ultrasound stone locking system. Journal of Endourology. 2015;**29**(11):1263-1269. DOI: 10.1089/end.2015.0175

[13] Owen NR, Bailey MR, Maxwell A, MacCongaghy B, Khokhlova TD, Crum LA. Vibroacoustography for targeting kidney stones during lithotripsy [abstract

#2aBB11]. The Journal of the Acoustical Society of America. 2004;**116**:2509

[14] Owen NR, Bailey MR, Crum LA, Sapozhnikov OA, Trusov LA. The use of resonant scattering to identify stone fracture in shock wave lithotripsy. The Journal of the Acoustical Society of America. 2007;**121**(1):EL41-EL47. DOI: 10.1121/1.2401266

[15] Leighton TG, Fedele F, Coleman AJ, McCarthy C, Ryves S, Hurrell AM, et al. A passive acoustic device for real-time monitoring of the efficacy of shockwave lithotripsy treatment. Ultrasound in Medicine & Biology. 2008;**34**(10):1651-1665. DOI: 10.1016/j.ultrasmedbio.2008.03.011

[16] Zeng G, Zhong W, Chaussy CG, Tiselius HG, Xu C, Turney B, et al. International Alliance of Urolithiasis guideline on shockwave lithotripsy. European Urology Focus. 2023;**9**(3):513-523. DOI: 10.1016/j.euf.2022.11.013

[17] Tran TY, McGillen K, Cone EB, Pareek G. Triple D score is a reportable predictor of shockwave lithotripsy stone-free rates. Journal of Endourology. 2015;**29**(2):226-230. DOI: 10.1089/end.2014.0212

[18] Abdelhamid M, Mosharafa AA, Ibrahim H, Selim HM, Hamed M, Elghoneimy MN, et al. A prospective evaluation of high-resolution CT parameters in predicting extracorporeal shockwave lithotripsy success for upper urinary tract calculi. Journal of Endourology. 2016;**30**(11):1227-1232. DOI: 10.1089/end.2016.0364

[19] Lingeman JE, Siegel YI, Steele B, Nyhuis AW, Woods JR. Management of lower pole nephrolithiasis: A critical analysis. The Journal of Urology. 1994;**151**(3):663-667. DOI: 10.1016/s0022-5347(17)35042-5

[20] Chaussy CG, Tiselius HG. How can and should we optimize extracorporeal shockwave lithotripsy? Urolithiasis. 2018;**46**(1):3-17. DOI: 10.1007/s00240-017-1020-z

[21] Koo V, Beattie I, Young M. Improved cost-effectiveness and efficiency with a slower shockwave delivery rate. BJU International. 2010;**105**(5):692-696. DOI: 10.1111/j.1464-410X.2009.08919.x

[22] Zeng T, Tiselius HG, Huang J, Deng T, Zeng G, Wu W. Effect of mechanical percussion combined with patient position change on the elimination of upper urinary stones/fragments: A systematic review and meta-analysis. Urolithiasis. 2020;**48**(2):95-102. DOI: 10.1007/s00240-019-01140-2

[23] Harper JD, Sorensen MD, Cunitz BW, Wang YN, Simon JC, Starr F, et al. Focused ultrasound to expel calculi from the kidney: Safety and efficacy of a clinical prototype device. The Journal of Urology. 2013;**190**(3):1090-1095. DOI: 10.1016/j.juro.2013.03.120

[24] Pishchalnikov YA, Neucks JS, VonDerHaar RJ, Pishchalnikova IV, Williams JC Jr, McAteer JA. Air pockets trapped during routine coupling in dry head lithotripsy can significantly decrease the delivery of shock wave energy. The Journal of Urology. 2006;**176**(6 Pt. 1):2706-2710. DOI: 10.1016/j.juro.2006.07.149

[25] Tailly GG, Tailly-Cusse MM. Optical coupling control: An important step toward better shockwave lithotripsy. Journal of Endourology. 2014;**28**(11):1368-1373. DOI: 10.1089/end.2014.0338

[26] Aboumarzouk OM, Hasan R, Tasleem A, Mariappan M, Hutton R, Fitzpatrick J, et al. Analgesia for patients

undergoing shockwave lithotripsy for urinary stones - A systematic review and meta-analysis. International Brazilian Journal of Urology. 2017;**43**(3):394-406. DOI: 10.1590/S1677-5538.IBJU.2016.0078

[27] Mancini JG, Neisius A, Smith N, Sankin G, Astroza GM, Lipkin ME, et al. Assessment of a modified acoustic lens for electromagnetic shock wave lithotripters in a swine model. The Journal of Urology. 2013;**190**(3):1096-1101. DOI: 10.1016/j.juro.2013.02.074

[28] Skuginna V, Nguyen DP, Seiler R, Kiss B, Thalmann GN, Roth B. Does stepwise voltage ramping protect the kidney from injury during extracorporeal shockwave lithotripsy? Results of a prospective randomized trial. European Urology. 2016;**69**(2):267-273. DOI: 10.1016/j.eururo.2015.06.017

[29] Lambert EH, Walsh R, Moreno MW, Gupta M. Effect of escalating versus fixed voltage treatment on stone comminution and renal injury during extracorporeal shock wave lithotripsy: A prospective randomized trial. The Journal of Urology. 2010;**183**(2):580-584. DOI: 10.1016/j.juro.2009.10.025

[30] Maxwell AD, Cunitz BW, Kreider W, Sapozhnikov OA, Hsi RS, Harper JD, et al. Fragmentation of urinary calculi in vitro by burst wave lithotripsy. The Journal of Urology. 2015;**193**(1):338-344. DOI: 10.1016/j.juro.2014.08.009

[31] Chen TT, Samson PC, Sorensen MD, Bailey MR. Burst wave lithotripsy and acoustic manipulation of stones. Current Opinion in Urology. 2020;**30**(2):149-156. DOI: 10.1097/MOU.0000000000000727

[32] Harper JD, Lingeman JE, Sweet RM, Metzler IS, Sunaryo PL, Williams JC Jr, et al. Fragmentation of stones by burst wave lithotripsy in the first 19 humans. The Journal of Urology. 2022;**207**(5):1067-1076. DOI: 10.1097/JU.0000000000002446

[33] Zwaschka TA, Ahn JS, Cunitz BW, Bailey MR, Dunmire B, Sorensen MD, et al. Combined burst wave lithotripsy and ultrasonic propulsion for improved urinary stone fragmentation. Journal of Endourology. 2018;**32**(4):344-349. DOI: 10.1089/end.2017.0675

Chapter 2

Role of ESWL in Era of Miniatured Endourological Modalities

Liaqat Ali, Faiza Hayat, Nasir Orakzai, Syeda Asiya Hassan and Danya Ali

Abstract

Extra corporeal shock wave lithotripsy (ESWL), being the first noninvasive stone treatment, was a landmark development. With its relatively good safety profile, cost effectiveness, and good results in certain types of stone management, it remained a prominent modality for three decades. However, because of the redefined indications for ESWL and the advancement of endourological equipment, its role has become limited. This chapter discusses the indications, advantages, limitations, and new developments of ESWL in this era of rapidly progressing minimally invasive stone surgeries.

Keywords: ESWL, urolithiasis, mini PCNL, ultra mini PCNL, RIRS

1. Introduction

> *"I will not cut, even for the stone..." Hippocrates*

As indicated in the Hippocrates oath, urolithiasis has affected mankind since ancient times, and it also reflects that its surgical management has always been challenging. ESWL invention in the 1980s thus straightaway attracted health care providers and patients towards this modality [1].

Despite the notable successes of newer surgical procedures to deal with renal tract stones, the ESWL, which uses ultrasonic shock waves, holds its place in urolithiasis treatment. It remains the first choice of therapy for relatively small, soft, and suitable-positioned stones [2].

ESWL's advantages:

1. It is relatively painless, and most patients can return home the same day.

2. It is a safe procedure with a low risk of complications.

3. It is a cost-effective procedure, making it more attractive in monetary terms for health care providers and patients too.

ESWL's disadvantages:

1. May not be as effective in treating relatively larger stones with increased density and in the lower pole of the kidneys.

2. There are chances of residual stone bulk, necessitating further treatment.

3. There is a small risk of complications, e.g., bleeding, infection, and renal parenchyma damage.

Overall, ESWL is a valuable tool in the treatment of stone disease, as long as the patient selection is correct [3–5].

2. The shockwave lithotripters

Prior to the development of ESWL in 1980, open stone surgery was the only treatment option for the management of renal tract stones, which were unlikely to pass spontaneously. Over the ensuing years, the modality was put to use mainly for upper renal tract stones [2].

The lithotripsy machines have four basic components:

1. Shockwave generator/energy source

2. Focusing system

3. Coupling mechanism

4. Localizing unit

With time, improvement in the lithotripters has mainly been focused on refining the shockwave generator. In the quest for the most effective lithotripter, there was a shift from electro-hydraulic to piezoelectric and finally to electromagnetic generators. The ultimate objective has been to have an ESWL system that is effective, results in minimal complications, and is cost-effective [2, 3].

3. The technical features of shockwave generators

3.1 Electrohydralic lithotripter

EHL was invented in Kyiv (Kiev) in 1954 and was used in the first model of ESWL in the 1980s by Dornier as HM3. The original method of shockwave is spark-gap technology. The energy that is generated by the spark gap results in vaporization bubbles that collapse and expand in a vicious cycle, and those bubbles strike and fragment the surface of stones (**Figure 1**).

3.2 Piezoelectric

The piezoelectric effect produces electricity via the application of mechanical stress. It was first described by the Curie brothers in 1880. The piezoelectric

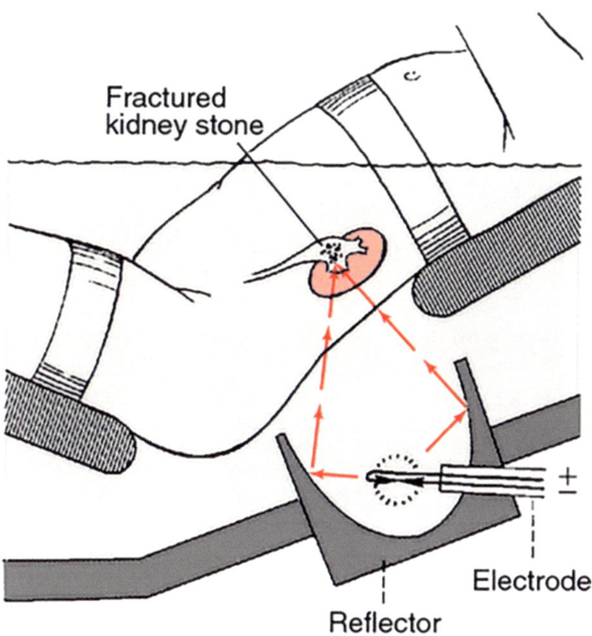

Figure 1.
Courtesy: ESWL. Electrically produced shock waves can fracture renal calculi. From Polaski and Tatro (1996).

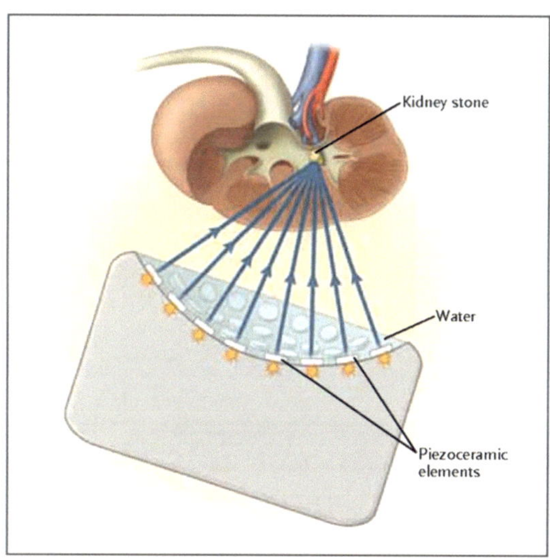

Figure 2.
Piezoceremic lithotripter. Courtesy: M. Pearle. Shock-wave lithotripsy for renal calculi. Published in the New England Journal of Medicine 2012.

lithotripter contains ceramic crystals in a water container. These ceramics are activated by high-frequency electrical pulses. These pulses result in the production of shockwaves for the fragmentation of stones (**Figure 2**).

Electromagnetic lithotripters are the latest generation of lithotripters. A high voltage is applied to an electromagnetic coil that creates high-frequency vibration

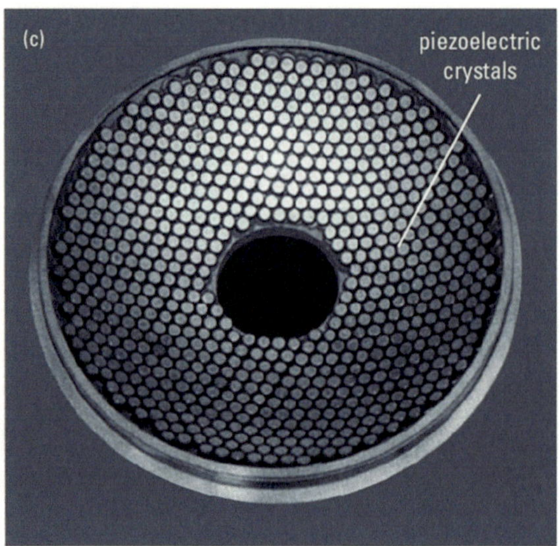

Figure 3.
Electromagnetic coil: this figure was uploaded by Achim M. Loske.

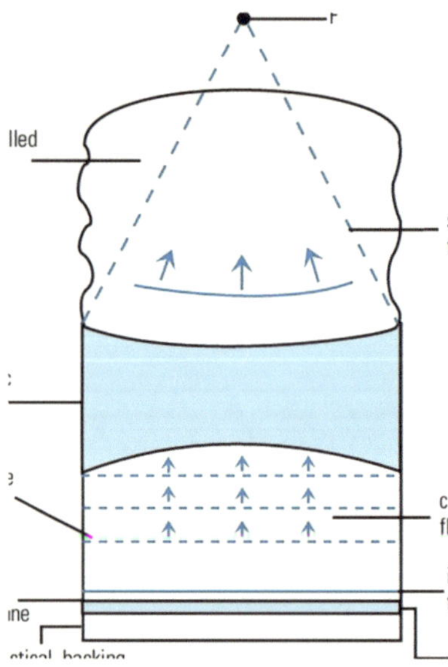

Figure 4.
Physics of electromagnetic lithotripsy: this figure was uploaded by Achim M. Loske.

in an attached metallic membrane. The oscillation is then transmitted to a wave-propagating medium to produce shockwaves (**Figures 3** and **4**).

There have been multiple studies comparing different machines for lithotripters. Sofras et al. conducted a comparative study with the Dornier HM3 and EDAP LT01 in 1000 patients. The stone-free rate (SFR) in 3 months was 87.5% vs. 90.4%. There was no significant difference for renal stones up to 1 cm [6]. The same findings were reported by Garber and Portis on HM3 lithotripters [7, 8]. A recent comparative trial among three lithotripters concluded that Dornier MPL 9000 resulted in superior treatment outcomes regarding stone-free rates and incidence of re-treatment when it was compared with Piezolith 2300 and Dornier Compact Delta [9]. All those comparisons have inherent flaws due to human, machine, and system biases [7]. Others compared different generations of machines. A comparative study of 13,864 calculi between an unmodified Dornier HM3 (5698 patients) and Medstone STS (8166 patients) found no complications or implications. This study showed SFR was 69.5% with the Dornier HM3 and 72.1% with the Medstone for single renal stones. While comparing the Piezolith 3000 to the previous Piezolith 2300 by matched-pair analysis, for single ureter stones, in 25 pairs [7], there were no differences in outcome.

Clayman defined the stone-free rate at a three-month interval better by the following formula: Effectiveness quotient = 100% stone free/100% stone free + % re-treatment + % auxiliary procedure %. Though this formula is very helpful in defining effectiveness, it still puzzles the researcher regarding clinically significant residual fragments [9].

4. Indications of ESWL in the twenty-first century

Recent literature contains important recommendations about ESWL concerning:

1. Predictors for stone fragmentation.

2. Predicting factors for treatment failure in lower pole and ureteric stones.

3. Contribution to the formulation of guidelines.

4. Maneuvers in procedures, e.g., slower rate and twin-pulse technique, for increasing efficacy and decreasing complications.

5. Comments on the potential role of medical treatment.

6. The role of ESWL in calyceal stones, clinically insignificant residual fragments, anomalous kidneys, obesity, and the ESWL pediatric population.

Before embarking on shockwave lithotripsy, the patient must be counseled for available alternate treatment options, allowing the patient to choose the mode of treatment. The clearance rate, the expected complications, and the procedure will be discussed in detail. A pre-procedure workup, like history, physical examinations, and biochemical profiles, is mandatory to exclude any contraindications to the treatment.

With the invention of advanced modalities like flexible ureteroscopy and mini percutaneous nephrolithotomy, shockwave lithotripsy is still being mentioned and recommended in European and American guidelines for small- to medium-sized suitable stones.

Several factors, such as stone burden, its location, the density in Hounsfield units (HU), pelvicalyceal anatomy, and the body mass index of the patient, determine the successful outcome of ESWL.

4.1 Stone size

Stones with a size less than 2 cm and favorable anatomy, such as upper midpole and pelvis stones, are more amenable to treatment.

However, in certain cases, where either the patient is not fit to undergo PCNL or is unwilling to have a surgical procedure, ESWL may be considered for stones a little larger than 2 cm. Obviously, in such patients, there are potential problems related to stone clearance and other complications, which are to be borne in mind.

4.2 Lower pole stones

Lower pole stones are difficult to clear with ESWL, but stones of appropriate size and low density may also be considered for ESWL. In addition, their clearance is also dependent on some anatomical features. The latter includes the lower pole-draining infundibular width, its length, and the infundibular pelvic angle. Stones with a size less than 1 cm have been reported to have a satisfactory clearance [3]. The details are shown in **Figure 5**.

In a randomized trial comparing the clearance of 14 mm lower pole calculus, the SFR was dramatically better with PCNL than ESWL, i.e., 95% vs. 37% [3]. Although stone-free rates are relatively lower in lower pole stones, tactics to facilitate fragments after shockwave lithotripsy are postural inversion, diuresis, and mechanical percussion, which can label 60% of these patients free of stone [5].

4.3 Ureteric stones

ESWL treatment of proximal ureteric stones between 1 cm and 1.5 cm has also been reported in the literature and guidelines. In a large randomized controlled study,

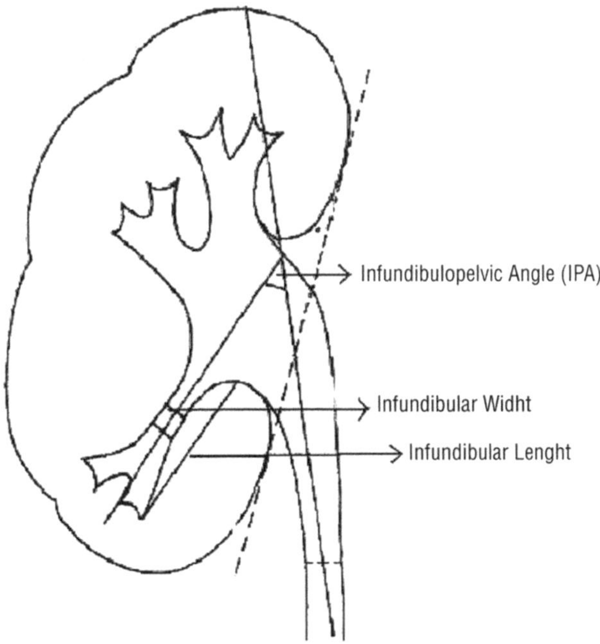

Figure 5.
Details of a anatomical predictive factors of Lower calyx for stone free rates in ESWL.

ureteroscopy showed a marginally improved outcome in terms of stone clearance; nevertheless, shockwave lithotripsy had better results in terms of health care costs [8].

4.4 In transplanted kidneys

Stones in transplanted kidneys have also been reported and successful, but caution must be exercised in dealing with such cases as patients are immunocompromised and anatomically different from the normal population. Distal patency for stone clearance post-procedure must be made ensured [10].

4.5 In bladder stones

Extracorporeal shockwave lithotripsy for bladder calculi has also been deemed safe and effective [11]. Bladder calculi are mobile and not ideal for ESWL; however, patients reluctant to undergo endoscopic procedures with stone sizes less than 2 cm can safely opt for ESWL.

4.6 Pre-ESWL Ureteric stents

The Pre-ESWL ureteric stent has been under a lot of controversy. For stones between 15 and 20 mm, a stent would prevent obstruction due to larger fragments. The stent itself requires the patient to undergo anesthesia and experience stent-related morbidity. Therefore, the placement of a stent is a personalized choice, keeping in mind the patient's condition, accessibility to the hospital in case of post-ESWL stone impaction, and other socioeconomic factors.

4.7 ESWL in obese patients

Controversy exists about the use of ESWL in obese patients as an important factor in predicting the outcome. Patients with a high body mass index, i.e., a BMI > 30 kg/m^2 are less likely to benefit from extracorporeal shockwave lithotripsy due to the increased skin-to-stone distance. A recent study proved the stone-free rates after 3 months in obese patients are 68% versus 80–85% in non-obese patients [5]. Obesity is also associated with a greater number of ESWL sessions. It is mentioned in the literature that patients with a waist circumference >10^2 cm require more than two sessions.

4.8 ESWL in the pediatric population

ESWL is still considered the most favorable therapeutic option in the pediatric population. ESWL is dramatically effective in stone fragmentation with low complication rates. Its effectiveness has been reported at a range of stone-free rates in children. For stones sized <20 mm, it's 67–93% in the short term and 57–92% in the long term. Stone-free rates in children after ESWL should be periodically assessed at a 3-month interval. A complete metabolic profile is mandatory for children with urolithiasis. Piezoelectric lithotripters are frequently mentioned with a lesser degree of pain in children. Our greatest invention is human curiosity. Minimal Access Surgery: Keeping in view the effectiveness quotient, the space of relative less clinical effectiveness of ESWL in terms of SFR was filled by the curiosity of scientists involved in making tools for minimal access surgery (MAS). In the second decade of the twenty-first century, MAS surpassed ESWL in clinical practice, evidence-based medical literature, and clinical effectiveness.

The journey of miniaturization from conventional PCNL to mini PCNL and ultra mini PCNL has so far taken a short stop on micro PCNL. All these miniaturizations have resulted in enhanced safety along with better stone fragmentation with the development of newer intracorporeal lithotripsy devices like lithoclast, trilogy, and holmium lasers. The development of effective flexible ureteroscopes with access sheaths has encouraged urologists to use mini PCNL in the supine position along with flexible URS in the same setting. All these developments in MAS, or natural orifice surgery, have studded the evidence-based medical literature. In a recently published meta-analysis by Kim et al. in 2020 [9], that, firstly, PCNL had the highest stone-free rates than others regardless of stone sizes, and RIRS showed higher stone-free rates than ESWL in <2 cm stones. Secondly, ancillary procedures were higher in ESWL than others. Finally, in stones <2 cm, the re-treatment rate of ESWL was higher. ESWL is still safer than other modalities, with a higher complication rate in PCNL than in URS and ESWL [9]. The 2023 EUA and AUA guidelines also endorse the better stone-free rates for endourological options of PCNL/URS in stone sizes above 20 mm, lower pole stones above 15 mm, and ureteric calculi. In upper ureteric calculi, the URS offers better SFR and ESWL a better safety profile. The safety profile of ESWL has also been enhanced by using losartan and selenium-based multivitamins. Other recent papers favor PCNL and URS as equally safe and effective in the low-volume disease of urolithiasis. A meta-analysis of 2927 patients with lower calyceal stones showed a decreased SFR for ESWL (52.9%) versus PCNL. The conclusion was that even stones of 11–20 mm are best treated by PCNL, with no difference in complication rates or quality of life [6, 9]. Thus, it is important to identify the patients likely to achieve failure in ESWL. With this, we can save the ESWL as one of the most effective modalities in the management of renal stones. For this purpose, the right patient selection should ensure the exclusion of persons with obesity, bleeding diathesis, failure of ESWL, complicated renal anatomy, hard stones on CT KUB, lower calyceal stones with unfavorable anatomy, struvite stones, and large stone burdens.

4.9 Safety profile of ESWL versus PCNL

Though literature suggests that PCNL and retrograde intra renal surgery (RIRS) are more effective in achieving stone-free rates in the management of urolithiasis than ESWL, however, ESWL still has, to its credit, a better safety profile than all sorts of percutaneous treatments. The complications of PCNL include intraoperative bleeding, hypotension, and postoperative hematuria. The need for blood transfusions in PCNL is about 3.5%. A recent meta-analysis published states that ESWL had lower complication rates than percutaneous nephrolithotomy ($p < 0.001$). However, there was no significant difference between complications of ESWL and RIRS [7–9].

4.10 ESWL, a landmark invention, from fading into oblivion

The first and foremost solution is that the established usefulness of ESWL must not be overlooked, and secondly, efforts to develop better-performing upgraded lithotripters must be hastened. In this regard, the new innovative technical developments are already underway.

The newer developments in SWL include twin-head and dual-pulse shock-wave generators; broad focus; low pressure systems; augmented coupling; self-operating location; and auditory tracking systems. The new developments, including evaluating lasers and histotripsy, have raised new hope for more effective ESWL. These innovations will contribute to a better SFR. As mentioned before, special emphasis should be drawn on attempting ESWL in obese patients, as it negatively affects the SFR not only for ESWL but also for endourological modalities [12].

It is worth mentioning that if the urologists get more familiar with the pathophysiology and physics of shock waves, much better results can be achieved in the future. This may lead to promoting the ESWL as one of the first lines of treatment in the management of urolithiasis in the era of miniature endoscopic equipment.

5. Summary

Despite all these years of the notable ESWL role and its exceptional importance as the only noninvasive stone treatment modality, the feeling of its diminishing importance is creeping in. This impression has developed due to the rapid development and success of MAS.

Nevertheless, with further refinements in the Lithotripters and attention paid to the correct patient selection for lithotripsy, ESWL still has a role in the treatment of certain renal or upper ureteric stones, especially in patients who cannot or prefer not to have stone surgery.

Ureteroscopy and PCNL offer higher success rates and greater versatility in treating larger or complex stones, but in terms of a better safety profile and cost effectiveness, ESWL still has an important place in the armamentarium for managing nephrolithiasis.

The European Union guideline suggests the use of ESWL or RIRS for the primary treatment of renal stones smaller than 2 cm and PCNL for stones larger than 2 cm. Although SFR is one of the essential points to consider when choosing among treatments, one also has to bear in mind the advantages and disadvantages of different methods of treatment when choosing the one that is most suited to that particular patient.

Author details

Liaqat Ali[1]*, Faiza Hayat[1], Nasir Orakzai[2], Syeda Asiya Hassan[1] and Danya Ali[3]

1 Institute of Kidney Diseases, HMC, Peshawar, Pakistan

2 Rehman Medical Institute, Peshawar, Pakistan

3 Peshawar Medical College, Peshawar, Pakistan

*Address all correspondence to: liaqat_99@yahoo.com

References

[1] Shafi H, Moazzami B, Pourghasem M, Kasaeian A. An overview of treatment options for urinary stones. Caspian Journal of Internal Medicine. 2016;**7**(1):1-6

[2] Petrides N, Ismail S, Anjum F, Sriprasad S. How to maximize the efficacy of shockwave lithotripsy. Turkish Journal of Urology. 2020;**46**(Suppl. 1):S19-S26. DOI: 10.5152/tud.2020.20441

[3] Albala DM, Assimos DG, Clayman RV, Denstedt JD, Grasso M, Gutierrez-Aceves J. Lower pole I: A prospective randomized trial of extracorporeal shock wave lithotripsy and percutaneous nephrostolithotomy for lower pole nephrolithiasis-initial results. The Journal of Urology. 2001;**166**:2072-2080

[4] Wiesenthal JD, Ghiculete D, Dah RJ, Pace KT. A comparison of treatment modalities for renal calculi between 100 and 300 mm^2: Are shockwave lithotripsy, ureteroscopy, and percutaneous nephrolithotomty equivalent? Journal of Endourology. 2011;**25**:481-485

[5] Pace KT, Tariq N, Dyer SJ, Weir MJ, Da Honey RJ. Mechanical percussion, inversion and diuresis for residual lower pole fragments after shock wave lithotripsy: A prospective, single blind, randomized controlled trial. The Journal of Urology. 2001;**166**:2065-2071

[6] Sofras F, Karayannis A, Kastriotis J, Vlassopoulos G, Dimopoulos C. Extracorporeal shockwave lithotripsy or extracorporeal piezoelectric lithotripsy? Comparison of costs and results. British Journal of Urology. 1991;**68**:15

[7] Graber SF, Danuser H, Hochreiter WW, Studer UE. A prospective randomized trial comparing 2 lithotriptors for stone disintegration and induced renal trauma. The Journal of Urology. 2003;**169**:54-57

[8] Argyropoulos AN, Tolley DA. Optimizing shock wave lithotripsy in the 21st century. European Urology. 2007;**52**:344-354

[9] Kim CH, Chung DY, Rha KH, Lee JY, Lee SH. Effectiveness of percutaneous nephrolithotomy, retrograde intrarenal surgery, and extracorporeal shock wave lithotripsy for treatment of renal stones: A systematic review and meta-analysis. Medicina. 2021;**57**:26. DOI: 10.3390/medicina57010026

[10] Challacombe B, Dasgupta P, Tiptaft R, Glass J, Koffman G, Goldsmith D. Multimodal management of urolithiasis in renal transplantation. BJU International. 2005;**96**:385-389

[11] Telha KA, Alkohlany K, Alnono I. Extracorporeal shockwave lithotripsy monotherapy for patiets with bladder stones. Arab Journal of Urology. 2016;**14**:207-210

[12] Bach C, Karaolides T, Buchholz N. Extracorporeal shock wave lithotripsy: What is new? Arab Journal of Urology. 2012;**10**:289-295

Section 2

Laser Lithotripsy

Chapter 3

Advanced Laser Mode for Ureteroscopic Lithotripsy Applications

Jian James Zhang

Abstract

The higher annual growth rate of kidney stone disease occurrence and the lower annual growth rate of practicing urologists require more efficient treatment tools. This chapter's research explores ways to increase laser lithotripsy stone ablation efficiency while reducing the stone retropulsion so that the stone procedure time can be effectively shortened. It covers the investigation of laser stone ablation threshold, ablation efficiency, retropulsion control, and the optimal dusting mode of a concept Holmium-doped yttrium aluminum garnet (Ho:YAG) laser with advanced tailored pulse technology to produce a high ablation rate and low retropulsion. Ho:YAG laser stone damage and recoil movement were investigated in vitro utilizing a tabletop model in a highly reproducible manner while evaluating the effects of several laser mode pulses. A thorough evaluation of the pseudo-optimal dusting mode's behavior (dusting rate and recoil movement) against a standard laser dusting mode was performed. The optimal dusting mode in this benchtop test model maintained a modest level of retropulsion while having a somewhat quick ablation rate. The transient pressure field measurement results of the standard and custom laser modes of a concept Ho: YAG laser are also included.

Keywords: laser lithotripsy, Ho:YAG, tailored laser pulse, dusting, ablation threshold, retropulsion, thulium fiber laser (TFL), transient pressure

1. Introduction

1.1 Kidney stones diseases

The kidney stone disease occurrence rate is 8.8% in the United States, with an annual growth rate of 5.5% [1]. However, according to the annual census of the American Urological Association (AUA), the annual growth rate of practicing urologists is 2.2%, and of the ratio of urologist-to-population is 1.8% [2]. The gap between disease treatment and the available physician requires efficient treatment tools.

The prevalence of kidney stone disease, urolithiasis, which is the production of hard tissue (stones) in the urinary tract as a result of oversaturated bodily fluids, has progressively increased in recent years. A decrease in urine volume (or water consumption), an increase in calcium oxalate/calcium phosphate secretion, a change in urine pH, and/or urinary tract infections (bacteria that produce urease) are the main reasons

IntechOpen

for stone formation [3–6]. According to estimates, 10–15% of cases occur in Western nations, and the recurrence rate can reach 50% [7–9]. And from 1995 to 2012, around 17 years, kidney stone prevalence increased by almost half, according to Charles D. Scales [10]. Due to factors such as population expansion, anticipated trends in obesity, and projected rises in diabetes, to name a few, the prevalence of urolithiasis has been increasing globally over the past few decades. By 2030, the annual cost of treating stone disease in the United States could exceed $5 billion (at 2014 pricing) [11, 12].

1.2 Advancement of treatment methods for urolithiasis

Even though percutaneous nephrolithotomy (PCNL) is also a "minimally invasive" procedure, the two treatments that are most frequently used in the US to treat patients with urinary calculi are shockwave lithotripsy (SWL) and ureteroscopic laser lithotripsy (URSL) [13, 14]. Due to a slightly faster recovery period and a higher stone-free percentage, URSL is currently the preferred urolithiasis treatment method [3].

Inspired by the theoretical research of Townes and Schawlow, Maiman [15] created the first laser device in 1960. In 1968, Mulvaney et al. [16] used quartz rods to carry the laser emission to the treatment target and documented the first disintegration of kidney calculus using a pulsed ruby laser (694 nm) in an in vitro experiment. After that, the pulsing second harmonic Nd:YAG laser (FREDDY), the pulsing dye-laser, and the triple doped yttrium aluminum garnet flash-lamp-pumped Ho:YAG laser were the three laser lithotripters that were clinically available [17–19]. Additionally, among all the commercially available lasers for lithotripsy, the flash-lamp-pumped Ho:YAG laser is the most effective and adaptable device when compared to nanosecond Nd:YAG lasers. All calculus compositions can be disintegrated by the Ho:YAG laser, and when compared to short-pulsed lasers, it causes less calculus recoil-movement (retropulsion) [20–24]. The Ho:YAG laser has long been the go-to lithotripter for the treatment of urinary calculus, having been developed in the 1990s. At a wavelength of 2.1 μm, it is a solid-state pulsed laser. Its broad margin of safety makes it perfect for lithotripsy in the urinary system because it is easily absorbed by water (26 cm^{-1} [25]) [26–28]. In addition to treating stone disease, it can be applied to soft tissue conditions such as removing urothelial tumors and curing urinary strictures. The prostate can be surgically removed using the high-powered variation (HoLEP). Thulium fiber laser technology has recently been investigated for future state of art laser lithotripsy [29, 30]. This cutting-edge method has a number of benefits that could push the limits of laser lithotripsy.

1.3 Challenges of laser lithotripsy (URSL)

Intracorporeal lithotripsy has been transformed by the use of medical lasers. The Ho:YAG laser and the more contemporary thulium fiber laser (TFL) are the main players of today, and pulse-modulation technologies can further modify how each of these lasers interacts with stones as well as the intermediary liquid medium. Ho:YAG laser lithotripsy primarily uses photothermal energy, with sonic emission having a minimal impact [31]. In other words, the Ho:YAG laser is photo-thermally restricted because its thermal diffusion time in water throughout its light propagation length is 286 ms [32], which is significantly longer than the laser pulse width (which is often less than a few milliseconds to a few hundred microseconds). Additionally, the Ho:YAG laser is neither photomechanically nor stress-confined in water due to the fact that the sonic diffusion time over the light propagation length is substantially shorter (0.267 μs) than the laser pulse width. Water strongly absorbs at the Ho:YAG

2.1 μm wavelength; hence, the amount of water in the calculus phantom was a factor in its ability to be removed from the sample [33, 34].

The stone disintegration speed, or ablation rate, is one of the essential factors determining laser effectiveness. A higher ablation rate can speed up the procedure, which means a shorter procedure time. And shorter procedure time is linked to less complication [35]. To reduce laser energy attenuation, the laser fiber should, in theory, be in direct contact with the stone. However, in fact, this is frequently not maintained consistently, and half or more of the pulsed laser energy may be transmitted while the fiber is more than 0.5 mm from the stone [36]. Ablation effectiveness is greatly affected if the fiber is not in contact with the stone.

Since its introduction into clinical practice, stone retropulsion has been a factor in intracorporeal laser lithotripsy. Early lasers, like the pulsed dye laser, functioned primarily by photoacoustic means by creating shockwaves that mechanically crushed stones [37, 38]. Stone retropulsion into the kidney increased risk and complexity via nephrostomy and antegrade ureteroscopy [39] and even signaled the end of the procedure due to the enormous quantities of kinetic energy involved and the lack of steerable flexible ureteroscopes [40]. As a result, retropulsion was often seen as a wholly negative phenomenon—a viewpoint that is still common today [41–43].

Urinary calculi absorb direct light, which raises the temperature of the exposed area above the ablation threshold and prompts the release of fragmented breakdown products. In addition, the creation of vapor bubbles and their subsequent collapse with shock-wave generation is caused by the absorption of laser energy by water between the fiber tip and calculus. The ablation threshold is one of the key variables in laser stone contact. According to the laser energy density, Richard L. Blackmon et al. [44] have investigated the ablation threshold for Ho: YAG and thulium fiber lasers (TFL). However, laser energy itself does not include the temporal information of the laser pulse. The peak power defines how fast the laser energy is delivered. Hence, a peak power density ablation threshold would be more broadly applicable.

Therefore, there are a few gaps in knowledge to be addressed, including peak power density ablation threshold, the transient pressure field of standard and advanced laser modes, and optimum laser dusting setting. In this chapter, we first measured the laser ablation threshold in terms of peak power density for the Bego stone phantom (15:3) with a fixed fiber and stone phantom setup [45]. Bego Stone is a reliable and consistent phantom material for lithotripsy study since it has physical properties matched with those of natural kidney stones of various chemical compositions [46]. The ablation volume is evaluated with direct laser-created crater measurement within the number of laser pulses below the crater volume saturation point. Then, we studied the transient pressure by the laser pulse in water by two types of hydrophones, optical and mechanical. The optimal dusting setting with the custom pulse modulation technology, developed considering the efficient use of laser energy to improve ablation efficiency with less retropulsion, is tested in a benchtop test model.

2. Experimental method and setup

2.1 Laser stone ablation threshold

In order to maintain consistency without human factor, the fiber and the stone phantom are fixed inside a water tank with the fiber tip in contact with the phantom as illustrated in **Figure 1**.

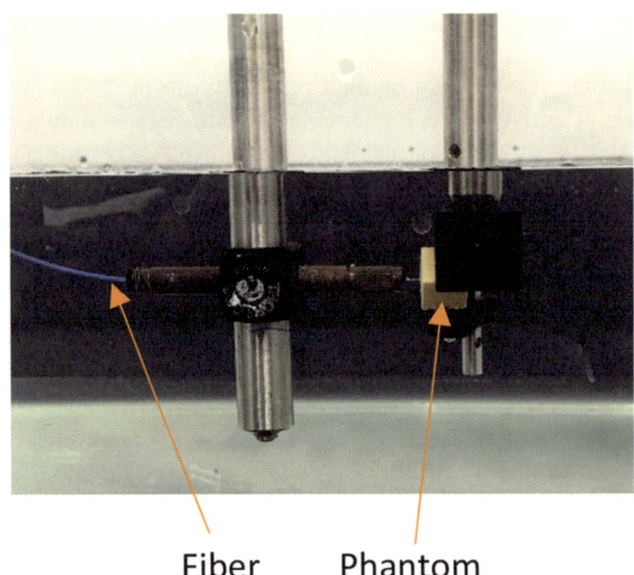

Figure 1.
The picture of the test setup.

Two Ho: YAG lasers that are readily accessible on the market were employed in this work as the laser pulse source. SureFlex™ fibers, Models S-LLF273 and S-LLF365, having core diameters of 273 and 365 μm, respectively, are the fibers employed in the experiment. The substance of the Bego stone (15:3) was used to create the calculus phantoms in the shape of a 10 mm cube. The Bego Stone was prepared with the lowest powder-to-water ratio 15:3 to simulate a natural kidney stone with the highest tensile strength [46]. The Ho: YAG lasers were used to ablate these stone phantoms at various peak power densities. The laser-induced crater volumes were assessed using a 3-D digital microscope (Keyence VHX-900F, Elmwood Park, NJ, USA), and the laser pulse width was determined using a 2 μm photodiode (Thorlabs DET10D). Since the pulse shape is not regular, we use the full width of 10% max as the pulse width definition. This allowed us to calculate the Bego stone phantoms' ablation threshold as a function of peak power density.

Figure 2 is a screenshot of the laser-induced crater by the 3-D digital microscope.

2.2 Transient pressure field measurement and retropulsion control

A prototype laser is used for the measurement, which can generate standard short pulse and two custom modes. SureFlex™ fiber, Model S-LLF365, having a core diameter of 365 μm, is the fiber employed in the experiment.

At the energies listed in **Table 1**, the prototype laser's three modes were tested using the default pulse width.

At least 40 pulses were included to produce every experimental data point, and the output is the highest hydrophone voltage signal. The largest standard deviation among the data gathered with the mechanical hydrophones was used in a 1-sample t-test. The estimated difference was 31%. The required sample size was determined to be n = 15 for the power of 95% at a significance level of = 0.05. For each of the 40 pulses, we record the highest voltage spike possible and also give the average of the Max.

DOI: http://dx.doi.org/10.5772/intechopen.1002881

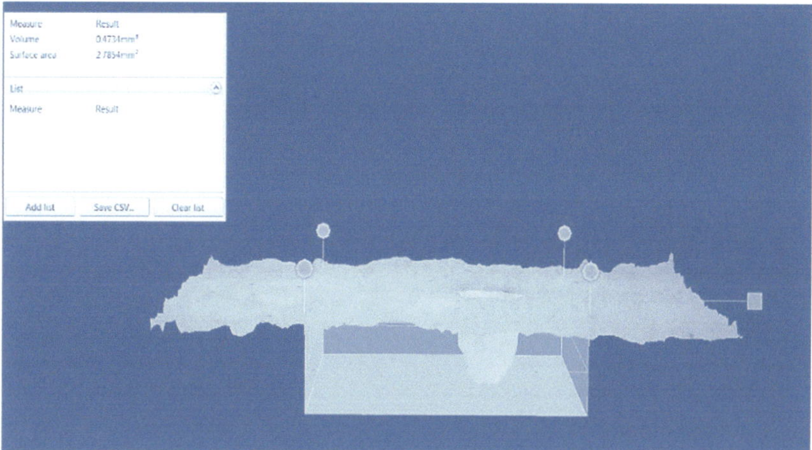

Figure 2.
A screenshot of the laser-induced crater by the 3-D digital microscope.

Laser mode	0.5 J	1 J	2 J	3 J
Standard-short	X	X	X	X
Fragmenting	—	X	X	X
Dusting	—	X	X	X

Table 1.
The list of energy settings of different laser modes.

Since the vapor bubble generated by the laser pulse is typically like an ellipsoid, we expect the transient pressure field to have a similar shape. Due to the fact that an ellipse is entirely determined by its major and minor axes, two measurement orientations—parallel and perpendicular—were investigated. The fiber and sensor tips were positioned in both cases (See **Figure 3**) 10 mm apart. The action center of the vapor bubble collapse, which normally takes place about 0.5 mm distant from the laser fiber tip, was aligned with the sensor at this distance, which reduced damage to the sensor tip from the incident shockwave.

2.3 The optimal dusting mode

Particularly when measuring retropulsion, it can be difficult to characterize the URS performance (ablation and retropulsion) in a single setup that can simulate the clinical condition [47–53]. Typically, the laser fiber is fixed during the test [4, 47, 54]. With a benchtop model previously developed by Sroka's group [4, 47], in vitro tests of Ho:YAG laser-induced stone ablation and retropulsion were carried out in this study. With the use of a hands-free setup and the measurement of the effects of several pulses that simulate a clinical setting, this test is extremely reproducible. Despite the fact that the stone moves during the test, causing the distance between the fiber tip and the stone to change and resulting in a decreased ablation rate being reported, this method is still effective for producing useful data about ablation and retropulsion for contrasting various laser modes. The list of elements in the experimental setup is described in **Table 2**. In **Figure 4**, the setup is shown. The composition of the Bego stone is 15:3 [46].

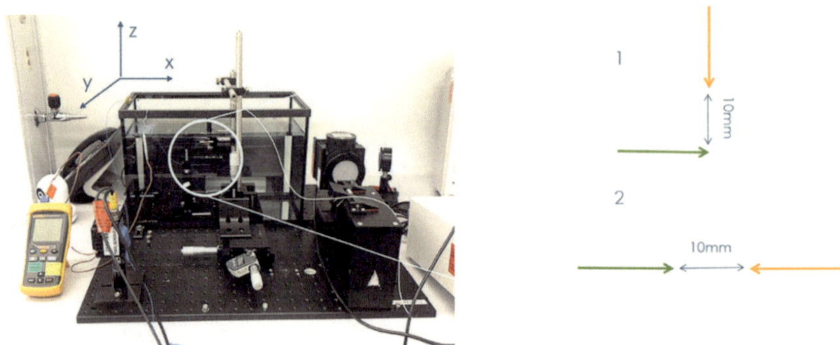

Figure 3.
Sensor to fiber orientation for the transient pressure field measurements.

Item	Description
Laser-1	Prototype Ho:YAG laser
Laser-2	Reference Ho:YAG laser
Laser fiber	365-µm S-LLF365 SureFlex™ Fiber (American Medical Systems, San Jose, CA, USA)
Stone phantom	BeGo (BEGO GmbH & Co. KG, Bremen, Germany)
Camera	Sony RX100 IV (Sony Corporation of America, NY, USA)
Balance scale	Sartorius Entris 224-1S (Sartorius Lab Instruments GmbH & Co. KG, Goettingen, Germany)
DOE programs	Design-Expert® (Stat-Ease, Inc., Minneapolis, MN 55413)

Table 2.
The list of components of the experimental setup.

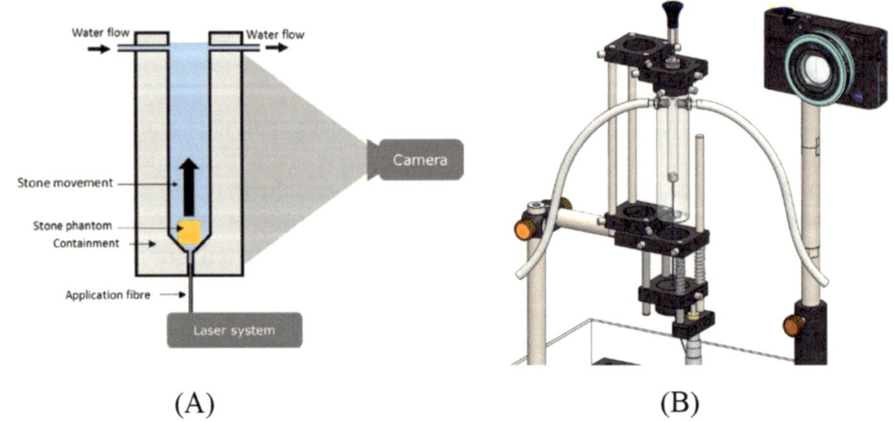

Figure 4.
Experimental setup (A) schematic diagram; (B) 3D rendering of the setup.

The speed at which the phantom moves vertically during the laser stone encounter is used to calculate the retropulsion. The setup's camera is a Sony RX100 IV, which can record the laser stone interaction video at 1000 frames per second. A MATLAB software is then used to process the footage.

Design-Expert® created the experiment with laser pulse energies of 0.2, 0.4, 0.6, 0.8, 1.2, and 1.5 J with frequencies of 5, 10, 15, 20, 30, and 40 Hz. with two replicate points, two lack-of-fit points, and randomized optimal (custom). The laser stone interaction test had a sample size of 14 and lasted 15 seconds for each laser setting. A P-value of 5% or less was regarded as statistically significant for all paired t-tests, which were all two-tailed tests.

3. Results

3.1 Laser stone ablation threshold

3.1.1 Saturation point evaluation

With fixed fiber and stone phantom, the laser-induced crater size will saturate after certain numbers of laser pulses due to the rapid decrease of laser ablation efficiency when the gap between the fiber tip and the stone increases. **Figure 5** is the crater volume saturation curve by two laser settings; each data point is the average of three measurements. The saturation happens after ~80 pulses.

3.1.2 Laser stone ablation threshold analysis

Figure 6 is laser stone ablation volume analysis curve by two laser types verses laser peak power density using pulse width definition of full width and 10%

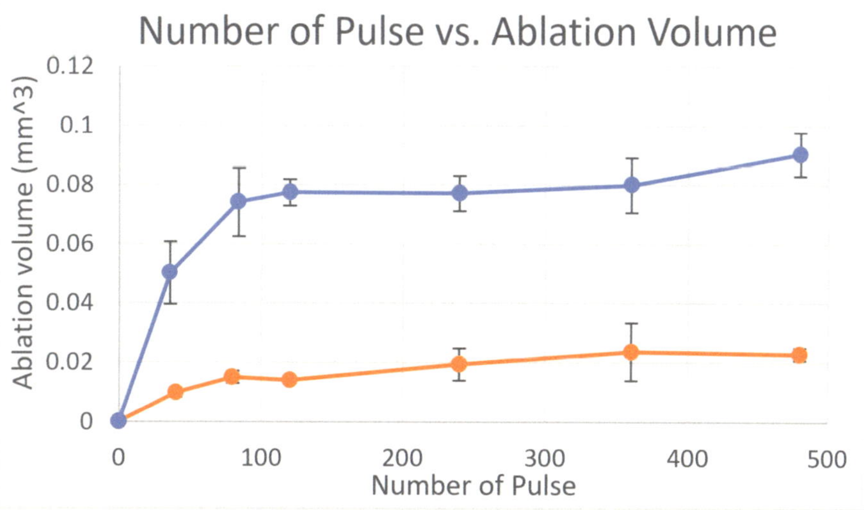

Figure 5.
Saturation point evaluation by laser 1 at 0.2 J 10 Hz (orange color curve) and laser 2 at 0.3 J 12 Hz (blue color curve).

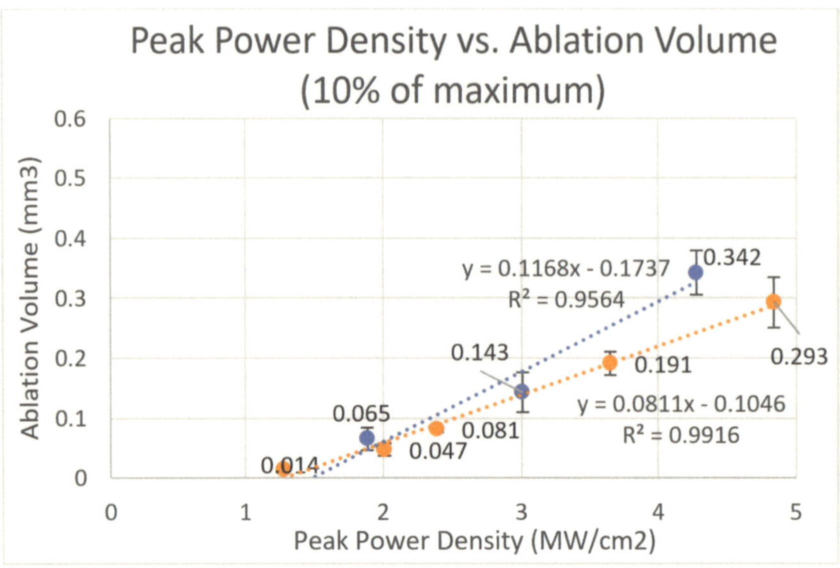

Figure 6.
The laser stone ablation volume analysis curve by two laser types (laser 1 in orange, and laser 2 in blue) versus laser peak power density using pulse width definition of full width and 10% maximum (FW10%M).

maximum (FW10%M). From the curves, we can calculate the laser ablation threshold in terms of peak power density is ~1.3 MW/cm^2 for laser 1, and ~ 1.5 MW/cm^2 for laser 2.

3.2 Transient pressure field measurement

For all of the measurements of transient pressure spikes, we employed the HNR-0500 hydrophone (the optical hydrophone was not suitable for this laser generated bubble transient measurement due to the optical effect of the bubble and its relative lower sensitivity). The majority of the spectral content is anticipated to be contained within 1 MHz, according to the Fourier Transform Analysis. The peak spectrum value can be used to calibrate the hydrophone's sensitivity. The measurement findings in terms of MPa are shown in **Tables 3** and **4**. Examples of the Transient Pressure Field Ellipsoids are shown in **Figure 7**.

3.3 The optimal dusting mode

Analysis of variance (ANOVA) of the tested data points, each of which represents the average of 14 measurements, is used by Design-Expert® to produce the response surfaces [55, 56]. The precise analytical formula for retropulsion and ablation in the optimal dusting mode is:

$$A_{\text{Optimal Dusting}}{}^{0.5} = 0.47 - 0.011\text{A} - 0.022\text{B} + 0.023\text{AB} + 0.0058BC \tag{1}$$

$$\left(\text{R}_{\text{Optimal Dusting}}\right) = 3.99 - 0.0025\,\text{A} + 0.091\,\text{B} + 0.014\,AB \tag{2}$$

Laser mode	Energy	Max_{Max} [MPa]		Min_{Min} [MPa]		Avg_{Avg} [MPa]	
		0°	90°	0°	90°	0°	90°
Prototype standard	0.5 J	2.2	2.9	0.3	0.2	0.8	1.0
	1 J	1.9	1.3	0.0	0.1	0.4	0.3
	2 J	2.7	0.9	0.1	0.1	0.8	0.3
	3 J	1.4	1.1	0.0	0.0	0.3	0.2
Prototype fragmenting	1 J	0.8	0.7	0.0	0.0	0.2	0.1
	2 J	1.6	1.2	0.1	0.1	0.4	0.3
	3 J	2.1	1.3	0.0	0.1	0.5	0.4
Prototype dusting	1 J	0.8	0.6	0.0	0.1	0.1	0.2
	2 J	0.5	0.6	0.0	0.0	0.1	0.1
	3 J	0.9	0.8	0.0	0.1	0.2	0.2

Table 3.
Measurement results of prototype laser.

Laser mode	Energy	Max_{Max} [MPa]		Min_{Min} [MPa]		Avg_{Avg} [MPa]	
		0°	90°	0°	90°	0°	90°
Reference standard short	0.5 J	2.1	1.6	0.6	0.5	1.2	1.0
	1 J	3.2	2.9	0.5	0.6	1.5	1.6
	2 J	3.7	5.2	0.7	0.6	1.6	2.2
	3 J	3.6	5.4	0.6	0.8	1.5	1.7

Table 4.
Measurement results of reference laser.

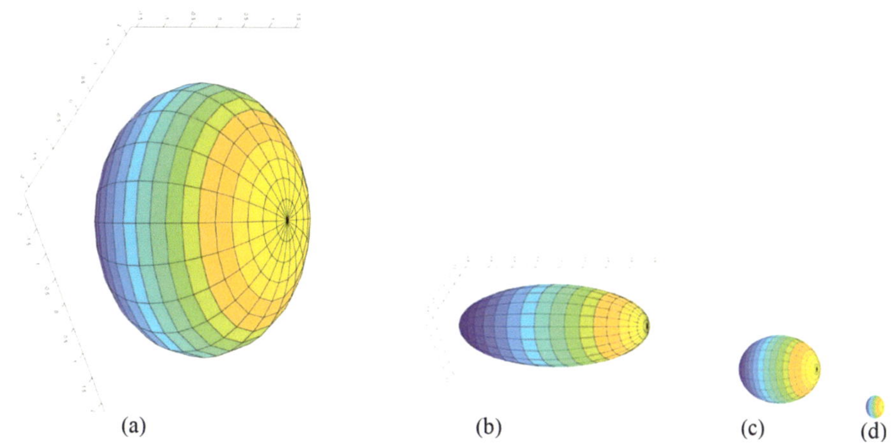

Figure 7.
Transient pressure field. (a) Reference laser 2 J (P_0/P_{90} = 1.6/2.2 MPa); (b) prototype laser standard short 2 J (P_0/P_{90} = 0.8/0.3 MPa); (c) prototype laser fragmenting 2 J (P_0/P_{90} = 0.4/0.3 MPa); (d) prototype laser dusting 2 J (P_0/P_{90} = 0.1/0.1 MPa).

A-Frequency (Hz), B-Energy (J), C-Pulse Width (ms), and $R_{Optimal\ Dusting}$-Retropulsion Velocity (mm/s) all contribute to optimal dusting.

The precise mathematical equation of the reference laser mode can be found in our earlier report in [57] as follows:

$$A_{Ref}^{0.5} = -0.28 + 0.00064A + 0.41B + 0.015AB \tag{3}$$

$$R_{Ref} = 49.1 + 0.28A + 43.8B \tag{4}$$

A-Frequency (Hz), B-Energy (J), A_{Ref}-Ablation rate (mg/s), R_{Ref}-Retropulsion Velocity (mm/s).

4. Discussion

4.1 Laser stone ablation threshold

The laser ablation threshold in terms of peak power density is a critical reference for laser lithotripsy efficacy. The lithotripsy laser peak power density needs to be more than the laser ablation threshold. Since it is a parameter of density, the laser delivery fiber also has a play. For a 365 μm core fiber, the laser peak power threshold is ~1.3 kW, and for a 230 μm core fiber, the peak power density threshold is ~0.5 kW, which is around the max peak power level of a commercially available Thulium fiber laser on the current market. Therefore, the current commercially available Thulium fiber laser may have a hard time breaking harder stones like brushite or calcium oxalate. And it can be mitigated by using a smaller core laser beam delivery fiber.

4.2 Transient pressure field measurement and retropulsion control

For stone retropulsion, peak power has a greater impact coefficient [58]. We must limit the transient pressure by lowering the peak power in order to reduce retropulsion while still exceeding the ablation threshold. The prototype Smart Modes' pulse modulation already contributes to this in several ways.

Our comprehension of the dynamic laser stone interaction during surgery is improved by bubble dynamics. A commercial Ho:YAG laser's bubble dynamics, including bubble size, shape, and energy delivery distance, were previously compared to those of the prototype laser. **Table 5** presents an overview of the information.

The speed of the laser energy injection is controlled by the laser pulse packet width. Except for the 0.5 J pulse, the prototype laser-generated bubble typically has an elongated form and is significantly smaller in height than the reference laser [59].

Power (W)	10	20	30	40
Optimal dusting mode	1 J 10 Hz	1 J 20 Hz	1 J 30 Hz	1 J 40 Hz
Referene dusting mode	0.25 J 40 Hz	0.5 J 40 Hz	0.6 J 50 Hz	0.8 J 50 Hz

Table 5.
The laser settings between the optimal dusting mode and dusting mode of the reference laser.

The lower transient pressure measurement result can be explained by the lesser height at 3 J compared to 2 J.

The spherical form of the 0.5 J bubble can be used to explain why the transient pressure value of the prototype laser's standard short mode at 0.5 J is greater than those of 1–3 J pulses. Due to its omnidirectional structure, the pressure peak at the bubble's collapse is very high. The vapor bubble's elongated/elliptical/rod shape at 1–3 J (caused by pulse modulation) disrupts the bubble's symmetry and lowers the transient peak pressure at the collapse.

A commercial Ho:YAG laser produces correspondingly huge vapor bubbles thanks to its high peak power and high energy pulses. Due to the omnidirectional nature of the vapor bubbles, a large portion of the energy injected is lost and not used for stone ablation. Longer water penetration tunnels and more focused vapor bubbles are produced by the prototype laser's Smart Modes. In non-contact laser lithotripsy treatments, dusting with a narrow and lengthy vapor bubble has the potential to increase efficiency by delivering the laser pulse farther.

4.3 The optimal dusting mode

The majority (>75%) of urinary tract calculi are thought to be calcium oxalate or mixed forms with calcium phosphate nuclei [60]. These most frequent stones are mostly caused by Randall plaques, which act as accretion sites and, thus, as a favored accumulation zone (seed) for precipitated solutes [61–66]. Urinary stones are known to have 100 different chemical components [5, 67]. The optimal lithotripsy laser dosimetry (setting), according to Sea J et al., relies on the particular case circumstance (calculus type, size, location, etc.), as well as the desired result [68]. There is not "one" optimal laser setting for URS, for this reason.

We must first specify the common laser parameters (power, energy, and frequency) used for URS in order to do our data analysis. Lower pulse energy (as low as 0.2 J) with a higher frequency is ideal for dusting needs since it produces significantly less retropulsion and smaller debris/remains [69]. High-power holmium settings (up to 40 W) fired in prolonged bursts with insufficient irrigation flow rates can result in high fluid temperatures in a laboratory "caliceal" model, despite the fact that higher power Ho:YAG lasers of up to 120 W are available for URS and the ablation rate is proportional to the laser power [70]. Higher irrigation flow rates, intermittent laser activation, and possibly chilled irrigation fluid are just a few of the ways urologists can control and reduce thermal effects now that they are aware of this risk [70].

The laser settings for the optimal dusting mode and the reference laser's dusting mode are listed in **Table 5**. The optimal dusting mode has a frequency range of 10–40 Hz and an energy level of 1 J. Use 40 or 50 Hz and low energy to calculate the average power level for the reference dusting mode.

The dusting modes of the reference laser and the prototype laser's ablation rate and retropulsion velocity are summarized in **Figures 8** and **9**. The average laser power is inversely correlated with the retropulsion velocity and ablation rate. The retropulsion velocity is more variable than the ablation rate, with a standard deviation that is 28% higher. The absolute value of the ablation rate will be lower than in studies with fixed fiber to stone distance [43, 54, 71, 72] since the stone phantom was not fixed during the test. Despite the drawbacks of (1) a reduced ablation rate due to stone movement; (2) retropulsion is a velocity that depends on the size of the phantom; the relative differences of the ablation rate and retropulsion velocity between the various

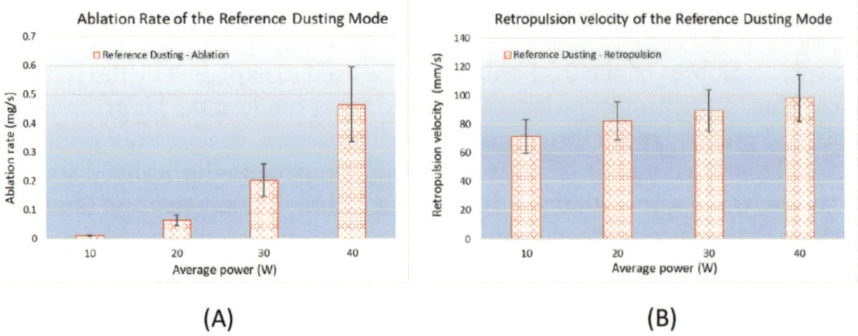

Figure 8.
Laser stone interaction results of the reference laser dusting mode. (A) Ablation rate vs. power; (B) retropulsion velocity vs. power.

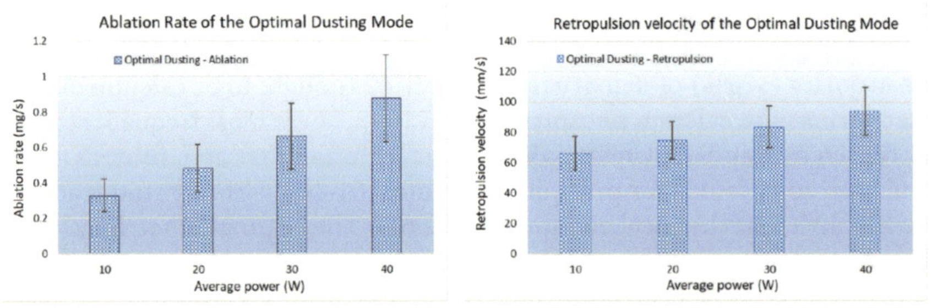

Figure 9.
Laser stone interaction results of the prototype laser dusting mode. (A) Ablation rate vs. power; (B) retropulsion velocity vs. power.

laser modes are comparable. The optimal dusting setting in this benchtop test model maintains a modest retropulsion while having a somewhat quick ablation rate.

5. Conclusions

In this chapter, we first measured the laser ablation threshold in terms of peak power density for the Bego stone phantom (15:3) was ~1.3 MW/cm^2. This is a critical reference for laser lithotripsy efficacy. Then we studied the transient pressure of the laser pulse in water. The study showed that the optical hydrophone's reduced sensitivity and distorted signal caused by the laser's generated vapor bubble make it ineffective for sensing laser-induced transient pressure in water. Mechanical hydrophones were used to measure and create the transient pressure field profiles. With the hydrophone ~10 mm away from the fiber tip, the reference laser's maximum transient pressure was 5.4 MPa and the prototype laser's was 2.9 MPa. The Standard mode of the prototype laser has the highest transient pressure, which is followed by the Fragmenting and Dusting modes.

In order to efficiently use laser energy to improve ablation efficiency with less retropulsion, we consider the ablation efficiency related to the laser ablation threshold and lower the transient pressure for retropulsion control. The optimal dusting setting with the custom pulse modulation technology in the benchtop test model maintains a modest retropulsion while having a quick ablation rate. All these studies' findings provide insights into future laser design to improve the efficiency, quality, and safety of lithotripsy procedures.

Acknowledgements

The authors thank the colleagues of Boston Scientific Corporation: Caroline Brial, Manjula Patel, John Goncalves, John Subasic, Jim Sarna, and Manuel Teixeira, Dongyul Chai, Gitanjali Multani, Brian Cheng, Xirong Yang, Baocheng Yang, David Jebbens, Ari Schwartz, Tram Vo, Trinh Pham, and Jasmine Cancino for laser test data gathering; Sean Curran, and Nicholas Nimchuk for their help on getting the software license of the Design-Expert® (DX10), as well as experimental data analysis, fitting, and optimization; and Sam Howard of Onda Corp. for setup and calibration of the hydrophones.

Disclaimer

The opinions expressed in this book chapter are solely those of the author and not necessarily those of Boston Scientific Corporation (BSC). BSC does not guarantee the accuracy or reliability of the information provided herein.

Author details

Jian James Zhang
Boston Scientific Corporation, Marlborough, MA, USA

*Address all correspondence to: james.zhang@bsci.com

References

[1] Scales CD Jr, Smith AC, Hanley JM, Saigal CS. Urologic diseases in America project. Prevalence of kidney stones in the United States. European Urology. 2012;**62**(1):160-165. DOI: 10.1016/j.eururo.2012.03.052

[2] AUA annual census. Practicing Urologists in the United States 2022 [Internet]. 2023. Available from: https://www.AUAnet.org/common/pdf/research/census/State-Urology-Workforce-Practice-US.pdf [Accessed: August 31, 2023]

[3] Yang C, Li S, Cui Y. Comparison of YAG laser lithotripsy and extracorporeal shock wave lithotripsy in treatment of ureteral calculi: A meta-analysis. Urologia Internationalis. 2017;**98**:373-381

[4] Bader MJ, Pongratz T, Khoder W, Stief CG, Herrmann T, Nagele U, et al. Impact of pulse duration on Ho:YAG laser lithotripsy: Fragmentation and dusting performance. World Journal of Urology. 2015;**33**:471-477

[5] Graham A, Luber S, Wolfson AB. Urolithiasis in the emergency department. Emergency Medicine Clinics of North America. 2011;**29**(3):519-538

[6] Türk C, Neisius A, Petřík A, Seitz C, Thomas K, Skolarikos A. EAU guidelines on urolithiasis 2018. In: European Association of Urology Guidelines. Presented at the EAU Annual Congress, Copenhagen. 2018th ed. Arnhem, The Netherlands: The European Association of Urology Guidelines Office; 2018

[7] Matlaga BR, Jansen JP, Meckley LM, Byrne TW, Lingeman JE. Economic outcomes of treatment for ureteral and renal stones: A systematic literature review. The Journal of Urology. 2012;**188**(8):449-454

[8] Rizvi SAH, Naqvi SAA, Hussain Z, Hashmi A, Hussain M, Zafar MN, et al. The management of stone disease. BJU International. 2002;**89**(Suppl. 1):62-68

[9] Tiselius HG. Epidemiology and medical management of stone disease. BJU International. 2003;**91**:758-767

[10] Scales CD Jr. Practice patterns in the management of urinary lithiasis. Current Urology Reports. 2013;**14**:154-157

[11] Turney BW, Reynard JM. The cost of stone surgery. European Urology. 2014;**66**:730-731

[12] Antonelli JA, Maalouf NM, Pearle MS, Lotan Y. Use of the National Health and Nutrition Examination Survey to calculate the impact of obesity and diabetes on cost and prevalence of urolithiasis in 2030. European Urology. 2014;**66**:724-729

[13] Pearle MS, Calhoun EA, Curhan GC. Urologic diseases of America project. Urologic diseases in America project: Urolithiasis. The Journal of Urology. 2005;**173**(3):848-857

[14] Seklehner S, Laudano MA, del Pizzo J, Chughtai B, Lee RK. Renal calculi: Trends in the utilization of shock-wave lithotripsy and ureteroscopy. The Canadian Journal of Urology. 2015;**22**(1):7627-7634

[15] Maiman TH. Ruby Laser Systems. US Patent 3,353,115. 1967

[16] Mulvaney WP, Beck CW. The laser beam in urology. The Journal of Urology. 1968;**99**:112-115

[17] Watson G, Smith N. Comparison of the pulsed dye and holmium lasers for stone fragmentation: In-vitro studies and clinical experience. Proceedings of SPIE. 1993;**1879**:139-142

[18] Tischer C, Koort HJ, Bazo A, Rasch R, Thiede C. Clinical experiences with a new frequency-doubled doublepulse Nd:YAG laser (FREDDY) for the treatment of urolithiasis. Proceedings of SPIE. 2002;**4609**:128-135

[19] Sayer J, Johnson DE, Price RE, Cromeens DM. Endoscopic laser fragmentation of ureteral calculi using the holmium:YAG. Proceedings of SPIE. 1993;**1879**:143-148

[20] Grasso M, Chalik Y. Principles and applications of laser lithotripsy: Experience with the holmium laser lithotrite. Journal of Clinical Laser Medicine & Surgery. 1998;**16**(1):3-7

[21] Marguet CG, Sung JC, Springhart WP, L'esperance JO, Zhou SL, Zhong P, et al. In vitro comparison of stone retropulsion and fragmentation of the frequency doubled, double pulse Nd:YAG laser and the holmium:YAG laser. The Journal of Urology. 2005;**173**(5):1797-1800

[22] Marks AJ, Teichman JMH. Lasers in clinical urology: State of the art and new horizons. World Journal of Urology. 2007;**25**(3):227-233

[23] Jansen ED, van Leeuwen TG, Motamedi M, Borst C, Welch AJ. Temperature dependence of the absorption coefficient of water for midinfrared laser radiation. Lasers in Surgery and Medicine. 1994;**14**(3):258-268

[24] Teichman JMH, Vassar GJ, Glickman RD. Holmium: Yttrium-aluminum-garnet lithotripsy efficiency varies with stone composition. Urology. 1998;**52**(3):392-397

[25] Grasso M. Experience with the holmium laser as an endoscopic lithotrite. Urology. 1996;**48**(2):199-206

[26] Chan KF, Vassar GJ, Pfefer TJ, et al. Holmium:YAG laser lithotripsy: A dominant photothermal ablative mechanism with chemical decomposition of urinary calculi. Lasers in Surgery and Medicine. 1999;**25**(1):22-37

[27] Pierre S, Preminger GM. Holmium laser for stone management. World Journal of Urology. 2007;**25**(3):235-239

[28] Teichman JMH, Rogenes VJ, McIver BJ, Harris JM. Holmium:Yttrium-aluminum-garnet laser cystolithotripsy of large bladder calculi. Urology. 1997;**50**(1):44-48

[29] Fried NM, Irby PB. Advances in laser technology and fiberoptic delivery systems in lithotripsy. Nature Reviews Urology. 2018;**15**:563-573

[30] Traxer O, Keller EX. Thulium fiber laser: The new player for kidney stone treatment? A comparison with holmium:YAG laser. World Journal of Urology. 2020;**38**(8):1883-1894

[31] Frenz M, Zweig AD, Romano V, Weber HP. Dynamics in laser cutting of soft media. Proceedings of SPIE. 1990;**1202**:22-33

[32] Niemz M. Laser-Tissue Interactions–Fundamentals and Applications. 2nd ed. Leipzig, Germany: Springer; 2002. p. 72. ISSN 1618-7210. ISBN 3-540-42763-5

[33] Rajabhandharaks D, Zhang JJ, Wang H, Xuan JR, Chia RWJ, Hasenberg T, et al. Dependence of water content in calculus phantom during Q-switched Tm:YAG laser lithotripsy. In:

Proc. SPIE 8565, Photonic Therapeutics and Diagnostics IX. 2013. 856519. Available from: SPIEDigitalLibrary.org

[34] Rajabhandharaks D, Zhang JJ, Wang H, Xuan JR, Chia RWJ, Hasenberg T, et al. Water content contribution in calculus phantomablation during Q-switched Tm:YAG laser lithotripsy. Journal of Biomedical Optics. 2015;**20**(12):128001

[35] Knipper S, Tiburtius C, Gross AJ, Netsch C. Is prolonged operation time a predictor for the occurrence of complications in ureteroscopy? Urologia Internationalis. 2015;**95**:33-37

[36] Aldoukhi AH, Hall TL, Ghani KR, Roberts WW. Strike rate: Analysis of laser fiber to stone distance during different modes of laser lithotripsy. Journal of Endourology. 2021;**35**:355-359

[37] Teng P, Nishioka N, Anderson RR, et al. Mechanisms of Laser-Induced Stone Ablation. In: Proc. SPIE 0712, Lasers in Medicine; 1987. p. 5. Available from: SPIEDigitalLibrary.org

[38] Thomas S, Pensel J, Engelhardt R, et al. The pulsed dye laser versus the Q-switched Nd:YAG laser in laser-induced shock-wave lithotripsy. Lasers in Surgery and Medicine. 1988;**8**(4):363-370. DOI: 10.1002/lsm.1900080405

[39] Grasso M, Shalaby M, el Akkad M, et al. Techniques in endoscopic lithotripsy using pulsed dye laser. Urology. 1991;**37**(2):138-144. DOI: 10.1016/0090-4295(91)80210-X

[40] Bolton DM, Peters JS, Costello AJ. Experience with the pulsed dye laser in management of ureteric calculi. The Australian and New Zealand Journal of Surgery. 1992;**62**(10):788-790. DOI: 10.1111/j.1445-2197.1992.tb06919.x

[41] Finley DS, Petersen J, Abdelshehid C, et al. Effect of holmium:YAG laser pulse width on lithotripsy retropulsion in vitro. Journal of Endourology. 2005;**19**(8):1041-1044. DOI: 10.1089/end.2005.19.1041

[42] Kamal W, Kallidonis P, Koukiou G, et al. Stone retropulsion with Ho: YAG and Tm: YAG lasers: A clinical practice-oriented experimental study. Journal of Endourology. 2016;**30**(11):1145-1149. DOI: 10.1089/end.2016.0212

[43] Wollin DA, Ackerman A, Yang C, et al. Variable pulse duration from a new holmium:YAG laser: The effect on stone comminution, fiber tip degradation, and retropulsion in a dusting model. Urology. 2017;**103**:47-51. DOI: 10.1016/j.urology.2017.01.007

[44] Blackmon RL, Irby PB, Fried NM. Journal of Biomedical Optics. 2011 Jul;**16**(7):071403. DOI: 10.1117/1.3564884

[45] Chai DY, Zhang JJ, Podana N, Xuan RJ, Hasenberg T, Harrah T. The study of Ho: YAG laser ablation thresholds of calculus phantom in terms of peak power density. In: Proc. SPIE 10852, Therapeutics and Diagnostics in Urology. 2019. 108520D. Available from: SPIEDigitalLibrary.org

[46] Esch E, Simmons WN, Sankin G, Cocks HF, Preminger GM, Zhong P. A simple method for fabricating artificial kidney stones of different physical properties. Urological Research. 2010;**38**(4):315-319

[47] Eisel M, Strobl S, Pongratz T, Strittmatter F, Sroka R. In vitro investigations of propulsion during laser lithotripsy using video tracking. Lasers in Surgery and Medicine. 2018;**50**:333-339

[48] Eisel M, Strobl S, Pongratz T, Strittmatter F, Sroka R.

Holmium:Yttrium-aluminum-garnet laser induced lithotripsy: In-vitro investigations on fragmentation, dusting, propulsion and fluorescence. Biomedical Optics Express. 2018;**9**(11):5115

[49] Zhang JJ, Rajabhandharaks D, Xuan RJ, Chia RWJ, Hasenberg TC. Characterization of calculus migration during Ho:YAG laser lithotripsy by high speed camera using suspended pendulum method. In: Proc. SPIE 8926, Photonic Therapeutics and Diagnostics X. 2014. 89261I-1-7. Available from: SPIEDigitalLibrary.org

[50] Kronenberg P, Traxer O. Update on lasers in urology 2014: Current assessment on holmium:Yttrium–aluminum–garnet (Ho:YAG) laser lithotripter settings and laser fibers. World Journal of Urology. 2015;**33**:463-469

[51] Hutchens TC, Gonzalez DA, Irby PB, Fried NM. Fiber optic muzzle brake tip for reducing fiber burnback and stone retropulsion during thulium fiber laser lithotripsy. Journal of Biomedical Optics. 2017;**22**(1):18001

[52] Sroka R, Haseke N, Pongratz T, Hecht V, Tilki D, Stief CG, et al. In vitro investigations of repulsion during laser lithotripsy using a pendulum setup. Lasers in Medical Science. 2012;**27**:637

[53] Zhang JJ, Rajabhandharaks D, Xuan RJ, Chia RWJ, Hasenberg TC. Calculus migration characterization during Ho:YAG laser lithotripsy by high-speed camera using suspended pendulum method. Lasers in Medical Science. 2017;**32**:1017-1021

[54] Kronenberg P, Traxer O. In vitro fragmentation efficiency of holmium: Yttrium–aluminum–garnet (YAG) laser lithotripsy: A comprehensive study encompassing different frequencies, pulse energies, total power levels and laser fibre diameters. BJU International. 2014;**114**(2):261-267

[55] Zhang JJ, Rutherford J, Solomon M, Cheng B, Xuan RJ, Gong J, et al. Numerical response surfaces of volume of ablation and retropulsion amplitude by settings of Ho:YAG laser lithotripter. Journal of Healthcare Engineering. 2018;**2018**:8261801. DOI: 10.1155/2018/8261801, 11 pages

[56] Zhang JJ, Rutherford J, Solomon M, Cheng B, Xuan JR, Gong J, et al. The study of laser pulse width on efficiency of Ho:YAG laser lithotripsy. In: Proc. SPIE 10038, Photonic Therapeutics and Diagnostics XIII. 2017. pp. 1-7. Available from: SPIEDigitalLibrary.org

[57] Zhang JJ, Chai D, Xuan RJ, Ray A, Hasenberg TC, Harrah T. In search of optimal settings for Ho:YAG laser lithotripsy to maximize the ablation rate, while minimizing the retropulsion. In: Proc. SPIE 11212, Therapeutics and Diagnostics in Urology. 2020. 1121204. Available from: SPIEDigitalLibrary.org

[58] Zhang JJ. In search of optimal laser settings for lithotripsy by numerical response surfaces of ablation and retropulsion. In: Kayaroganam P, editor. Response Surface Methodology in Engineering Science. London, United Kingdom. 2021. Online ISBN: 978-1-83968-918-5, Print ISBN: 978-953-51 3459 6 (Aug 23, 2021). DOI: 10.5772/intechopen.96271

[59] Zhang JJ, Xuan JR, Yu H, Devincentis D. Study of cavitation bubble dynamics during Ho:YAG laser lithotripsy by high-speed camera. Proceedings of SPIE. 2016;**9689**:E-1-E-7

[60] Chan KF, Pfefer TJ, Teichman JMH, Welch AJ. A perspective on laser lithotripsy: The fragmentation processes. Journal of Endourology. 2001;**15**(3):257-273

[61] Coe FL, Evan AP, Worcester EM, Lingeman JE. Three pathways for human kidney stone formation. Urological Research. 2010;**38**:147-160

[62] Kuo RL, Lingeman JE, Evan AP, Paterson RF, Parks JH, Bledsoe SB, et al. Urine calcium and volume predict coverage of renal papilla by Randall's plaque. Kidney International. 2003;**64**:2150-2154

[63] Kim SC, Coe FL, Tinmouth WW, Kuo RL, Paterson RF, Parks JH, et al. Stone formation is proportional to papillary surface coverage by Randall's plaque. The Journal of Urology. 2005;**173**:117-119

[64] Miller NL, Gillen DL, Williams JC Jr, Evan AP, Bledsoe SB, Coe FL, et al. A formal test of the hypothesis that idiopathic calcium oxalate stones grow on Randall's plaque. BJU International. 2009;**103**:966-971

[65] Miller NL, Williams JC Jr, Evan AP, Bledsoe SB, Coe FL, Worcester EM, et al. In idiopathic calcium oxalate stone-formers, unattached stones show evidence of having originated as attached stones on Randall's plaque. BJU International. 2010;**105**:242-245

[66] Low RK, Stoller ML. Endoscopic mapping of renal papillae for Randall's plaques in patients with urinary stone disease. The Journal of Urology. 1997;**158**:2062-2064

[67] Khan A. Prevalence, pathophysiological mechanisms and factors affecting urolithiasis. International Urology and Nephrology. 2018;**50**:799-806

[68] Sea J, Jonat LM, Chew BH, et al. Optimal power settings for holmium:YAG lithotripsy. The Journal of Urology. 2012;**187**(3):914-919

[69] Aldoukhi AH, Roberts WW, Hall TL, Ghani KR. Holmium laser lithotripsy in the new stone age: Dust or bust? Frontiers in Surgery. 2017;**4**:57

[70] Aldoukhi AH, Ghani KR, Hall TL, Roberts WW. Thermal response to high-power holmium laser lithotripsy. Journal of Endourology. 2017;**31**(12):1308-1312

[71] Aldoukhi AH, Roberts WW, Hall TL, Ghani KR. Watch your distance: The role of laser fiber working distance on fragmentation when altering pulse width or modulation. Journal of Endourology. 2019;**33**(2):120-126. DOI: 10.1089/end.2018.0572

[72] Elhilali MM, Badaan S, Ibrahim A, Andonian S. Use of the Moses technology to improve holmium laser lithotripsy outcomes: A preclinical study. Journal of Endourology. 2017;**31**(6):598-604

Chapter 4

Perspective Chapter: Clinical Indications for the Use of Laser in Urolithiasis

Victor Enrique Corona-Montes, Vanessa Júarez-Cataneo and Juan Eduardo Sánchez-Núñez

Abstract

Current technology has improved the modalities of intra-corporeal lithotripsy, including: ultrasound and ballistic, combined with different laser energies useful in the most important procedures for resolving urinary system stones. Nowadays, the amount of lasers and their availability has grown considerably, lasers like Holmium:Yttrium-Aluminum-Garnet (Ho:YAG) and Thulium Fiber Laser (TFL) are the most effective and safest alternatives for lithotripsy in several types of endo urological strategies for lithotripsy. The selection of appropriate laser energy is crucial to optimize the usefulness in the management of urinary tract stones and it depends on the clinical indications validated for the International Urolithiasis Alliance based in technology but also in principles of management from the reported outcomes based in the expertise of several endo urological surgeons. Both, Ho:YAG laser and TFL are effective systems of fragmentation in retrograde intrarenal surgery (RIRS) and percutaneous nephrolitotomy (PNL), even in the miniaturized percutaneous tracts enhanced with suction. Comparative with other types of lithotripsy, they have the same stone-free rates, low complication indexes, and optimal surgical operative times. Urologists must be familiar of with the properties of each laser to get the best surgical outcomes for the benefits of their patients. The present chapter will describe the clinical indications and the adequate use of laser fibers.

Keywords: lithotripsy, laser, holmium, Thulium, intra renal surgery

1. Introduction

Urolithiasis is the more often benign pathology in urology. Its incidence can be higher in some specific climes and countries. Nowadays there is an increase in innovations and technology for the treatment of kidney stones. Lithotripsy is a minimally invasive procedure used to treat calculi localized in the urinary tract like the kidney, the ureter, and the bladder, those stones need different management to be treated basically with some principles according to several factors like size, localization. Lithotripsy actually has some elements and different technical aspects, and technologies like the administration of energy directly to the stone in order to get fragmentation or dusting of the calculi to free the urinary tract from them [1, 2].

Urologists account for several modalities of intracorporeal lithotripsy, including: ultrasound, ballistic, combined, and laser energy useful in the most important treatments of stone diseases. Some approaches are percutaneous nephrolithotomy (PNL) and retrograde intrarenal surgery (RIRS). More recently, in the context of complex or Staghorn calculi, we have a new approach that mix both techniques named endoscopic combined intrarenal surgery (ECIRS) [3, 4].

However, this has been the most widely used option for intracorporeal management of urinary calculi due to its effectiveness regardless of the stone composition and its high lithiasic clearance capacity, therefore is a growing interest in the development of new laser energies [5–8].

Laser energies in recent years have offerred very new modalities. Thulium laser which has exceptional results in stone fragmentation and seems to be promising given that it offers good clinical results compared to Ho:YAG laser [9–11].

2. Laser lithotripsy types

In the modern era of lithotripsy, we have two effective modalities for stone clearance. These are Holmium laser and Thulium laser, which are the result of technological development in order to improve efficiency and safety [9].

2.1 Holmium:YAG

The Holmium:YAG is the most used laser for lithotripsy. This conventional laser can be used for retrograde intrarenal surgery. When used as a high-power laser in RIRS could be associated with a decrease in the operating room time and a higher Stone Free Rate (SFR) specifically when compared to the lower-power devices.

When it is used with lower frequency and a combination of higher energy and shorter pulse duration again higher frequency, lower energy, and longer pulse duration, the improvement reflects an ability to generate dusting.

The Holmium laser is a well-defined and extensively source of energy for lithotripsy. It has an excellent capability of fragmentation instead of stone type and density, and its low tissue penetration allow a good safety margin for surrounding tissue and a low thermal effect for the contiguous epithelium. Several studies, including meta-analysis, had not demonstrated differences between stone-free rates compared with Thulium Fiber Laser and the postoperative complications between both groups are very similar [12–14].

2.2 Tulium

The Tulium laser has become a relative new but effective technology and safe. It allows the use of high frequencies and reduction in the retropulsion offering efficiency in ablation. Both lasers need the urologist consideration to be aware of their thermal effects, as they also have adequate irrigation and working space.

The Thulium Fiber Laser is a recent innovative laser technology that seems particularly promising in stone treatment. There is a necessity of more studies to define the future of lithotripsy through the good results TFL is achieving [15].

Ho:YAG laser lithotripsy offers the same stone-free rates compared to other fragmentation modalities (ultrasonic, pneumatic, and combined) as it is highly effective in terms of fragmentation regardless of stone composition. In contrast, it requires more surgery because the stone clearance time is longer compared to other modalities. In the literature, a lower rate of complications associated with bleeding is reported with laser lithotripsy (Ho:YAG) compared with other fragmentation modalities [16].

So, the election between laser modalities will depend on the surgeon's expertise and clinical setting, the continuous development of those, will offer a broad spectrum of lithotripsy modalities which will be a milestone in stone management [13].

3. Current indications

Current indications for intracorporeal lithotripsy are indistinct between laser energy used (Ho:YAG vs. Thulium). Even, in the management of urinary stones in children we have the same indications and energy applications.

There exist a global effort to standardize the clinical diagnosis and management of urinary tract stones. Several organizations, including the American Urological Association (AUA), European Association of Urology (EAU), and National Institute for Health and Care Excellence (NICE) have worked to enhance clinical guidelines for a better approach to urolithiasis [2, 4, 17].

Consider for asymptomatic renal stones in adults and children, watchful waiting (WW) approach if the stones are smaller than 5 mm and if the stone is larger than 5 mm but the patient or their family carers agrees to watchful waiting (WW) [16, 18].

4. In the case of symptomatic stones, consider the following approaches

4.1 Retrograde intrarenal surgery (RIRS)

Retrograde intrarenal surgery has been a very useful minimally invasive approach for ureteral stones. Some of the following are clinical indications according to the size stone. The proximal ureteral calculi with a diameter less than 20 mm (LE:1, GR:A), intra-renal calculi with a diameter less than 20 mm (LE:1, GR:A), intra-renal or ureteral calculi in the proximal third of the ureter greater than 20 mm when there is a contraindication for percutaneous nephrolithotomy (*LE:2, GR:B).

Retrograde surgery for intra-renal or proximal ureteral calculi with a diameter less than 20 mm with laser fragmentation offers better success rates in a single procedure and lower rates of reoperation compared with extracorporeal lithotripsy [2, 18].

4.2 Percutaneous nephrolithotomy (PNL)

Since the percutaneous nephrolithotomy was born in 1979. It came as an innovative and precise minimally invasive procedure for greater stone diameter and at the beginning for lower calix localization. The main indications are in the kidney stones with a diameter greater than or equal to 20 mm in diameter (*LE:1, GR:A), and for difficult access upper urinary tract calculi (*LE: 2, GR: B), those can include inferior caliceal location, infundibular narrowing, narrow infundibulum-pelvic angle, and anatomical renal abnormalities.

Percutaneous nephrolithotomy (PNL) is the treatment modality for calculi larger than 20 mm or staghorn calculi. In those cases in which the PNL has a failure the use of extracorporeal lithotripsy or intrarenal retrograde surgery is recommended (LE: 2, GR: B).

4.3 Endoscopic combined intrarenal surgery (ECIRS)

There is always the possibility of performing a combined endoscopic procedure, is necessary to consider if we are facing a calculi with complex configuration, greater than 2 cm, when: (*LE: 2, GR: B), in those cases where the NLPC is not feasible, and if retrograde intrarenal surgery as monotherapy is not enough.

The need for re-intervention due to the high stone volume or the high probability of residual stones after a single procedure is an indication for a combined approach [18] (**Figures 1–3**).

5. Complications

Associate complications to the RIRS procedures and to the use of lasers can be bleeding, ureteric perforation or avulsion, arterio-venous fistula, perirenal hematomas, infections.

The risk of bleeding when present is due to an injury generally self-limited or due to a perforation of the ureter or collecting system by insertion of fibers, guidewires,

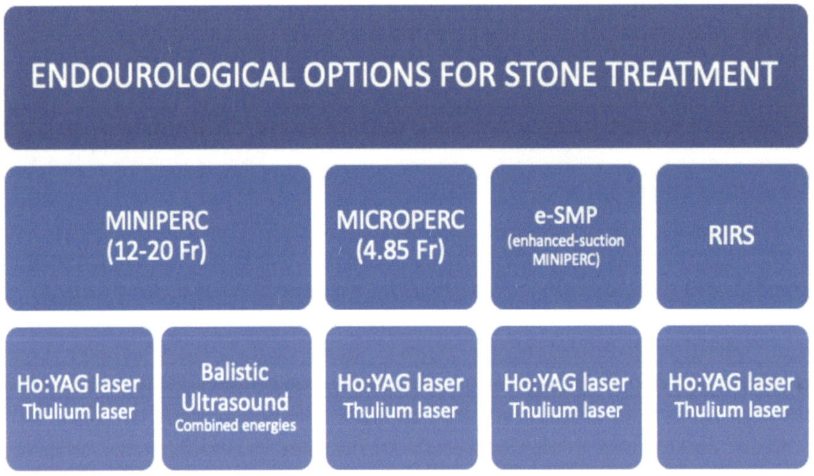

Figure 1.
*Modalities of energy usefulness in different endourological approach to urinary tract stones. *LE, level of evidence; GR, grade recommendation.*

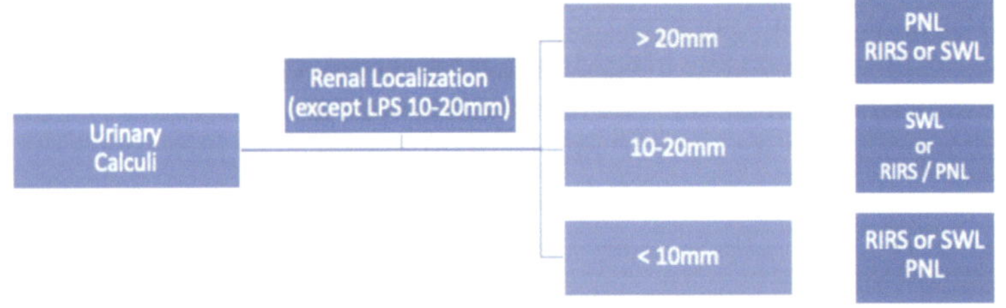

Figure 2.
*Summary recommendations by international Urolithiasis Alliance for urinary tract stones considering size and location [16, 18]. *PNL, percutaneous nepholithrotomy; RIRS, retrograde intrarenal surgery; SWL, shock wave lithotripsy; LPS, lower pole stone.*

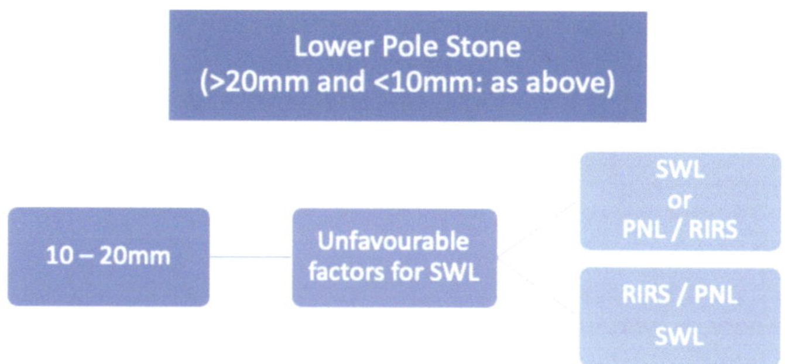

Figure 3.
*Summary recommendations by international Urolithiasis Alliance for urinary tract stones considering size and location [16, 18]. *PNL, percutaneous nephrolithotomy; RIRS, retrograde intrarenal surgery; SWL, shock wave lithotripsy; LPS, lower pole stone.*

catheters creating a perforation or avulsion, special patient conditions like anticoagulation therapy or change in decompression after high intrarenal pressure.

Secondary to the use of energy lasers inadvertent thermal injury can also produce bleeding that generally is self-limited, however, wall injuries are properly described in the endoscopic classification system [19].

The main reasons to develop an infection are infection stone, size of burden stone, prolonged operating time, and forced irrigation, all of them can be prevented with adequate use of operative intrarenal pressure, shorter time of operation, proper antibiotic prophylaxis, and use of a Foley catheter.

Complications in PCNL have a bigger range in Clavien-Dindo classification, they are clearly lower with mini PCNL, the first is the bleeding present as hematuria according to not significant or even to avoid the proper view in the field, causing even incidence of transfusion or embolization can be required previous angiography control [16].

Describe risk factors for bleeding such as the urinary tract infection, infected stones, comorbidities as diabetes mellitus, associated to the puncture technique or anatomical aspects like lower kidneys or solitary kidney, and during the intervention as long operation time for the procedure.

Avoiding infections with adequate antibiotic previous therapy is required, in specific cases, a culture can be obtained intraoperative. The risk of a systemic inflammatory response syndrome (SIRS), urosepsis can be present, especially associated with the following risk factors preoperative positive urine test, recurrent infection, kind of stone as staghorn calculi, and during procedure associated to prolonged operative time and high renal pelvic pressure. Treatment must be implemented promptly and should be appropriate antibiotics, in some cases resuscitation support and intensive unit care maybe required.

Urinary extravasation occurs when a high intra-renal pressure is maintained, torquing the nephroscope, perforation of calyceal system clinically observed as abdominal distention, airway resistance and oxygen desaturation, considered to stop the procedure to place a nephrostomy and ureteral stent should be performed, an ultrasound evaluation to drain the peritoneal effusion by puncturing [16].

Injury to organs can be present according to the level of puncture, pleural, hydrothorax, hemothorax, pneumothorax a drainage tube could be necessary, liver or spleen are also probably present in supra-costal punctures, management can be conservative or urgent laparotomy's.

Large bowel injury will be demonstrated by ultra-sonography guidance, CT scan or fistulography. The result will be an urgent laparotomy in front of an acute peritonitis, percutaneous colostomy, bowel rest, intravenous broad-spectrum, and parenteral nutrition will be recommended for the management [16].

6. Discussion

When and how to treat urinary stones depends on the size, location, and severity of the clinical manifestations.

It is important to remember that urinary calculi smaller than or equal to 4 mm with expulsive therapy in a period of 14–21 days, will achieve successful spontaneous passage in up to 80% of patients [2].

There are cases of asymptomatic renal ureteral lithiasis, according to current literature, up to 50% of them will develop some type of clinical manifestation within 5 years, so it is important to treat with the intention of preventing complications associated with them [1].

The need for intra-corporeal treatment has favored the development of laser technology for fragmentation or pulverization in situ. Over time, the modalities are becoming more efficient, safer, and accessible to the general population.

The advent of the Ho:YAG laser has favored better perioperative results in terms of stone-free rates and the number of procedures required for total stone clearance [7].

The characteristics of the laser fiber allow better synergy with flexible and semirigid ureteroscopes. The imminent need and trend for the miniaturization of percutaneous tracts will improve the development of better laser technologies to continue their usefulness in fragmentation matters [20–22].

Technology is now moving forward to develop laser innovations related to calculi fragmentation and pulverization: energy delivery systems, pulse and frequency applications, fiber quality and tip-shape novel designs, etc. Certainly, these innovations will contribute to the best endourological surgery performance to achieve better efficiency in the management of urinary tract stones [23].

The International Urolithiasis Alliance has a social commitment in order to create optimal clinical guidelines that will be actualized within an interval of two years because all the surgical systems, energies and devices development, etc. [16, 18].

7. Conclusions

We are in an era of a well-developed laser energies, which are capable of solving any kind of urinary stones. The clinical results demonstrate excellent stone-free rates after one procedure, a few necessities of re-intervention, safer procedures, and optimal operative times.

The selection of appropriate laser energy is crucial to optimize the efficiency and safety during endourological procedures.

The Ho:YAG laser is the most effective system for flexible ureteroscopic lithotripsy and the most useful for fragmentation through miniaturized percutaneous tracts with suction.

The Thulium laser is a new fragmentation modality. Its versatility (high frequencies and low retropulsion) seems to offer a promising outlook, but studies are needed to confirm these advantages in terms of lithotripsy.

Urologists must be acquainted with the properties of each laser to get the best surgical outcomes for the benefit of our patients.

Acknowledgements

Thanks to collaborative group and special thanks to them who provided linguistic revision.

Conflict of interest

The authors declare no conflict of interest.

Notes/thanks/other declarations

None.

Nomenclature

PNL	percutaneous nephrolithotomy
RIRS	retrograde intrarenal surgery
ECIRS	endoscopic combined intrarenal surgery
Ho:YAG	Holmium:Yttrium-Aluminum-Garnet
AUA	American Urological Association
EAU	European Association of Urology
NICE	National Institute for Health and Care Excellence
IUA	International Urolithiasis Alliance
WW	watchful waiting
LE	level of evidence
GR	grade of recommendation
LPS	lower pole stone
TFL	Thulium Fiber Laser
SIRS	systemic inflammatory response syndrome

Author details

Victor Enrique Corona-Montes[1,2]*, Vanessa Júarez-Cataneo[2] and Juan Eduardo Sánchez-Núñez[1,2]

1 Department of Urology, American British Cowdray, Centro Médico (A.B.C.), México City, México

2 Urology Department, Hospital General de México "Dr. Eduardo Liceaga", México City, México

*Address all correspondence to: urocorona@hotmail.com

References

[1] Hughes T, Ho HC, Pietropaolo A, Somani BK. Guideline of guidelines for kidney and bladder stones. Turkish Journal of Urology. 2020;**46**(Suppl 1):S104-S112

[2] Türk C, Petřík A, Sarica K, Seitz C, Skolarikos A, Straub M, et al. EAU guidelines on diagnosis and conservative management of urolithiasis. European Journal of Urology. 2016;**69**(3):468-474

[3] EAU Guidelines on Diagnosis and Conservative Management of Urolithiasis – PubMed [Internet]. [citado 1 de junio de 2023]. Disponible en: https://pubmed.ncbi.nlm.nih.gov/26318710/

[4] Kidney Stones: Surgical Management Guideline – American Urological Association [Internet]. [citado 1 de junio de 2023]. Disponible en: https://www.auanet.org/guidelines-and-quality/guidelines/kidney-stones-surgical-management-guideline

[5] Ashmawy A, Khedr M, Saad IR, Zamel S, Kassem A. Laser lithotripsy using dusting technique (low energy, high frequency) for symptomatic upper urinary tract stones. African Journal of Urology. 2021;**27**(1):155

[6] Strittmatter F, Eisel M, Brinkmann R, Cordes J, Lange B, Sroka R. Laser-induced lithotripsy: A review, insight into laboratory work, and lessons learned. Transl Biophotonics. 2020;**2**(1-2):e201900029

[7] Tzelves L, Somani B, Berdempes M, Markopoulos T, Skolarikos A. Basic and advanced technological evolution of laser lithotripsy over the past decade: An educational review by the European Society of Urotechnology Section of the European Association of Urology. Turkish Journal of Urology. 2021;**47**(3):183-192

[8] Laser Lithotripsy – an overview | ScienceDirect Topics [Internet]. [citado 1 de junio de 2023]. Disponible en: https://www.sciencedirect.com/topics/medicine-and-dentistry/laser-lithotripsy

[9] Denstedt J, Gabrigna Berto FC. Thulium fiber laser lithotripsy: Is it living up to the hype? Asian Journal of Urology. 2022;**2022**:S2214

[10] Gonzalez-Cuenca E, Razvi H. Thulium fiber laser: Game changer or marketing hype? Revista Mexicana de Urología. 2023;**2023**:83. Disponible en: https://revistamexicanadeurologia.org.mx/index.php/rmu/article/view/1013

[11] Ryan JR, Nguyen MH, Linscott JA, Nowicki SW, James E, Jumper BM, et al. Ureteroscopy with thulium fiber laser lithotripsy results in shorter operating times and large cost savings. World Journal of Urology. 2022;**40**(8):2077-2082

[12] Kim HJ, Ghani KR. Which is the best laser for lithotripsy? Holmium laser. European Journal of Urology Open Science. 2022;**44**:27-29

[13] Liang H, Liang L, Yu Y, Huang B, Chen J, Wang C, et al. Thermal effect of holmium laser during ureteroscopic lithotripsy. BMC Urology. 2020;**20**(1):69

[14] Chua ME, Bobrowski A, Ahmad I, Kim JK, Silangcruz JM, Rickard M, et al. Thulium fibre laser vs holmium: Yttrium-aluminium-garnet laser lithotripsy for urolithiasis: meta-analysis of clinical studies. BJU International. 2023;**131**(4):383-394

[15] Ulvik O, Aesoy MS, Juliebo-Jones P, Gjengsto P, Beisland C. Thulium fibre laser versus holmium:YAG for Ureteroscopic lithotripsy: Outcomes from a prospective randomised clinical trial. European Urology. 2022;**82**(1):73-79

[16] Zeng G, Zhong W, Mazzon G, Choong S, Pearle M, Agrawal M, et al. International Alliance of Urolithiasis (IAU) Guideline on percutaneous nephrolithotomy. Minerva Urology and Nephrology. December 2022;**74**(6):653-668. DOI: 10.23736/S2724-6051.22.04752-8

[17] Singh A, Shah M, Hameed BMZ, Singh A, Shah M, Hameed BMZ. Guideline Based Algorithmic Approach for the Management of Renal and Ureteric Calculi. IntechOpen; 2022. Disponible en: https://www.intechopen.com/online-first/84098

[18] Zeng G, Traxer O, Zhong W, Osther P, Pearle MS, Preminger GM, et al. International Alliance of Urolithiasis guideline on retrograde intrarenal surgery. BJU International. 2023;**131**(2):153-164

[19] Traxer O, Thomas A. Prospective evaluation and classification of ureteral wall injuries resulting from insertion of a ureteral access sheath during retrograde intrarenal surgery. The Journal of Urology. 2013;**189**(580):4

[20] Gao X, Wang W, Peng L, Di X, Xiao K, Chen J, et al. Comparison of micro-percutaneous and mini-percutaneous nephrolithotomy in the treatment of renal stones: A systematic review and meta-analysis. Frontier in Surgery. 2021;**8**:743017

[21] Zhu W, Huang Z, Zeng G. Miniaturization in percutaneous nephrolithotomy: What is new? Asian J Urol [Internet]. 7 de febrero de 2023 [citado 31 de mayo de 2023]. 2023. Disponible en: https://www.sciencedirect.com/science/article/pii/S2214388223000243

[22] Ganpule AP, Vijayakumar M, Malpani A, Desai MR. Percutaneous nephrolithotomy (PCNL) a critical review. International Journal of Surgery. 2016;**36**:660-664

[23] Sabler IM, Katafigiotis I, Gofrit ON, Duvdevani M. Present indications and techniques of percutaneous nephrolithotomy: What the future holds? Asian Journal of Urology. 2018;**5**(4):287-294

Section 3

Pneumatic and Ultrasound Lithotripsy and Paediatric Stone Management

Chapter 5

New Technologies in Ultrasonic and Pneumatic Lithotripsy

Charalambos Kypraios, Ioannis Xoxakos, Ntiela Ntonta and Ioannis Efthimiou

Abstract

Background: Ultrasonic and pneumatic lithotripters are the gold standard for percutaneous nephrolithotripsy. The goal of this chapter is to help the reader become more familiar with the newer lithotripters and to critically select the best available lithotripsy device for each situation. Methods: A literature search was performed to identify all types of older and newer generation ultrasonic and ballistic lithotripters. Physics, characteristics, efficacy, and safety are discussed. Results: Newer dual lithotripters are more effective and allow disruption of stones both in the laboratory and clinical trials. CyberWandTM and Lithoclast Select lithotripters have similar stone disintegration rates in percutaneous nephrolithotripsy for stones >2 cm. UrerTron has a very rapid stone clearance rate, especially for hard stones, with no difference in stone clearance rates or need for secondary procedures. Lithoclast® Trilogy demonstrated superior stone clearance time compared to ShockPulse™ and Swiss Lithoclast® Select (Master) with high stone volume clearance rates in both standard and mini PCNL with a mean stone-free rate of 83%. However, more recent data have shown that neither lithotripsy device offers a clinically meaningful advantage over older generation devices. Conclusion: All the new lithotripsy devices have an excellent safety profile. They do not appear to be any more effective than the older generation devices. The advantages, disadvantages, and costs of each type of intracorporeal lithotripter must be considered when choosing a treatment modality for a particular case.

Keywords: endourology, ultrasonic, pneumatic, lithotripsy, combination

1. Introduction

Endourology is now the main player in the treatment of urinary stone disease. Intracorporeal lithotripsy is the cornerstone of modern endourology. It provides safe, effective, and reliable disintegration of urinary lithiasis. This advantage has translated into improved stone-free rates, reduced morbidity, and faster patient recovery. Technological advances in this field have led to the acceptance of endourology by urologists worldwide. Percutaneous nephrolithotripsy is generally considered the treatment of choice for stones 2 cm in diameter, staghorn calculi, or after failure of other endourologic procedures. It is a well-established procedure with stone-free rates exceeding 80%. Despite the high cure rates, there is a push for better results with an even faster procedure to reduce surgical time, especially for hard and large stones. In the last decade, there has been a trend toward combined lithotripsy procedures to overcome this handicap.

In this chapter, we first discuss the history, physics, and mechanics of ultrasonic and ballistic lithotripters. We then introduce the major players, from older to newer devices: the Swiss LithoClast® Select lithotripter, CyberWandTM, UreTron, ShockPulse SETM, and EMS Lithoclast® Trilogy. Key features, efficacy, and safety are discussed with a brief review of the current literature. The goal of this chapter is to help the reader become more familiar with the newer lithotripters and to critically select the best available lithotripsy device for the situation.

2. History of rigid lithotripsy

Ultrasonic vibration energy is more than 70 years old. The idea of using ultrasonic vibrational energy to disintegrate urinary calculi originated with Mulvaney, who tested the first model of lithotripsy in 1953 [1]. Successful in vivo ultrasonic lithotripsy was performed much later in 1970 by Terhorst [Terhorst], who used the energy to treat bladder stones [2]. Later in the 1970s, Marberger and Alken reported the first successful cases of percutaneous nephrolithotripsy (PCNL) with ultrasound in humans [3]. In 1993, pneumatic lithotripsy with the Swiss Lithoclast appeared in the field of intracorporeal lithotripsy [4]. A year later, a new device for ballistic lithotripsy with electrokinetic energy appeared on the market and the first series appeared in the international literature [5].

Since then, the innovation technology allowed the combination of both energies in the same device for better disintegration of the stones [6, 7].

3. Physics and properties of ultrasonic lithotripsy

Ultrasonic waves have an acoustic frequency that is inaudible to humans. Ultrasonic lithotripsy is based on the generation of ultrasound waves with a specific frequency of about 23–25 kHz. First, electric current is transmitted from an ultrasound generator to a handpiece transducer via a coaxial cable. The handpiece consists of piezoceramic elements and a longitudinal steel probe, which is adjusted at the distal tip of the probe. Activation of the device via a foot pedal causes excitation of the piezoceramic elements to produce acoustic waves at the specified frequency. The probe begins to vibrate in the longitudinal and transverse directions. When the probe comes into contact with a stone, the acoustic energy is transferred to the stone and the stone decomposes. The probe is usually hollow, and the back part of the handpiece is also connected to an aspirator to suck out small fragments and debris. If the probe is small in diameter, the suction cannot be used. Smaller probes are suitable for ureteric stone lithotripsy and larger ones for bladder and kidney stones.

Tissue changes are minimal and occur only after direct contact with the urothelium [8, 9]. Direct application of the ultrasound probe to the urothelial wall may cause epithelial abrasions and hemorrhagic edema of the lamina propria, which disappear after about a week [10]. A main advantage of ultrasonic lithotripsy is that it has a large safety margin even with a contact time of more than a few seconds with a minor force against the ureteral wall [11].

In PCNL, ultrasonic lithotripsy is performed by gently pressing the stone against the renal pelvis and rotating the probe against the stone to pulverize it by creating craters on it. This maneuver is repeated several times on the stone surface. The stone eventually weakens and disintegrates into smaller particles that are removed from the field by suction.

The probes are solid or hollow and vary in size from 2.5–5 Fr. They need a straight working channel. If they are twisted or bent at the insertion point of the working probe, ultrasonic energy is lost and heat is generated. Eventually, the probe becomes fatigued and may break at the junction with the handpiece.

Ultrasonic lithotripters successfully disintegrate soft stones, but hard stones, such as calcium oxalate monohydrate, brushite, and cystine are disintegrated less efficiently. Although the tip of the probe heats up during the procedure, this increase in temperature appears to be of limited clinical significance. The rise in temperature is limited to as low as 1.4°C, especially if adequate fluid irrigation in the surgical field of at least 30 ml/min is provided [12]. It provides excellent fragmentation and stone-free rates of 97% and 94%, respectively, with a low complication rate [13].

4. Physics and properties of pneumatic lithotripsy

The working principle of pneumatic lithotripsy is based on the momentum theorem. It is an analog of Newton's cradle that allows the impact of one ball to remove another, and so on. A metal projectile was forced with a precision of one micrometer at high speed. When the projectile hits the probe installed in the handpiece, a shockwave is transmitted through the probe to the calculus [14].

In ballistic lithotripsy, energy is transmitted by the forward movement of a projectile, such as a jackhammer. The handpiece device receives energy from either an electromagnetic field or compressed air from the wall, and pneumatic lithotripters have a frequency of 12 Hz and receive compressed air at 3 atm. Electrokinetic lithotripters have a slightly higher frequency—15–30 Hz—and receive energy from the electromagnetic field. The different mechanical properties of the metal probe and stone lead to fast and effective lithotripsy. Proper fixation of the stone between the urothelium and probe eases the transmission of energy to the stone. Like ultrasound probes, ballistic probes also require rigid and straight working channels. Bowing of the probe results in considerable energy loss. Ballistic lithotripters can break hard stones regardless of their composition; however, they cannot produce fragments smaller than 4 mm [10]. This property makes ballistic lithotripsy useful for kidney and bladder stones and less useful for ureteric stones. The probe sizes are 0.8, 2.5, and 3.8 mm.

It has a good safety profile, with no thermal effects on the surrounding tissues and low maintenance costs [15]. Drawbacks include the risk of fragment migration, use of an offset semirigid ureteroscope, and the need for a basket or graspers to remove the fragments [13, 15]. In addition, in the presence of impacted stones in the case of lithotripsy in a narrow space, for example, a narrowed calyceal neck hemorrhage is less likely because of the mechanical impact of the road and repeated friction between the students, and because of the original collection system, this humoral loses the vision of the film.

The Cook StoneBreaker LMA™ is another type of portable ballistic lithotripter that does not require an external source of compressed air and uses prefilled cartridges filled with CO2. Each cartridge can deliver about 100 shocks. In a comparative study with Swiss Lithoclast, the device showed easier setup, use, and faster stone fragmentation [16]. A similar portable ballistic lithotripter is the EMS Swiss LithoBreaker, an electrokinetic lithotripter with a rechargeable battery. It delivers a single continuous shot at 3 Hz and a source capacity of up to 3.000 impulses. The probe sizes are 2.4–6 Fr. A single in vitro study showed decreased effectiveness of the device in a percutaneous model on a Bego Stone compared to a portable pneumatic device [17].

Regarding the biological effects on tissues, it seems that Lithoclast behaves in a manner similar to that of ultrasound lithotripters. Histologically, it induces minimal lesions consisting of a reduction in cell layers, epithelial detachment, and mild parietal edema [10].

The fragmentation and stone-free rates for both electrokinetic and pneumatic lithotripters are similar and are between 84 and 97.5% and 70–95%, respectively [13].

5. Operating principles of combination technologies in ultrasonic and pneumatic lithotripsy

The combination of both energies has the advantages of both energies. On the one hand, constant emission of ultrasonic energy allows for fine fragmentation and dusting of stones, whereas intermittent ballistic shocks allow for the powerful and coarse fragmentation of large and hard stones. Thus, it could be assumed that initially, the hard parts of a stone break up with the ballistic part to bigger fragments, and as the lithotripsy advances, the ultrasonic component leads to pulverization of the small and short fragments of the stone. Simultaneous suction allows continuous removal of debris and even larger stone fragments, depending on the size of the probe. All combinations of older and newer lithotripters are presented in **Table 1**.

Type	Probe		Energy	Company
The Swiss LithoClast® Select Lithotripter	two probes	reusable	ultrasonic and pneumatic energy	EMS S.A., Switzerland/Boston Scientific, USA
CyberWandTM	two probes	reusable	ultrasonic waves in two different frequencies	Olympus, Tokyo, Japan
UreTron	one probe	reusable	ultrasonic frequency control technology	Richard Wolf
ShockPulse SETM	one probe	reusable/ single use	constant ultrasonic wave energy lithotripter with intermittent shock wave (ballistic/ mechanical) energy	Olympus
Swiss Lithoclast® Trilogy	one probe	single use	ultrasound and electromagnetic ballistic energy	EMS S.A., Switzerland

Table 1.
Newer generation and combination lithotripers.

6. Types of new lithotripters

6.1 Swiss LithoClast® select lithotripter (EMS S.A., Switzerland/Boston Scientific, USA)

The Swiss LithoClast® Select Lithotripter device is a two-probe dual-modality. This device also allows simultaneous transmission of ultrasonic and pneumatic energy to the stones when it is used with a special handpiece of the Vario device. Each type of energy can also be used separately for each of the two probes. It also allows for the same session to switch from only ultrasonic energy to both modes of energy. It also allows suction. Occasionally, malfunction of the device can occur with clogging of the probe. The main advantage of the combination of pneumatic and ultrasonic lithotripters is that they can disintegrate and clear stones at a more effective and rapid rate with slightly improved stone-free rates [9, 18, 19].

6.2 CyberWand™ (Olympus, Tokyo, Japan)

CyberWand™ is an electromechanical device that is capable of fragmenting and aspirating calculi. The handpiece has an ultrasonic transducer containing a piezoelectric element, which is driven by a generator operating at 20–22 kHz. This is a dual-ultrasonic lithotripter. It has two separate ultrasonic probes that vibrate at two different frequencies, high and low. The outer probe, 3.75 mm in diameter, vibrates at one kHz and is designed for breaking smaller stones. The inner probe is designed for larger stones with a 2.77 mm and vibrates at 21 kHz with a 2.1 mm hollow inner lumen. Its efficacy is thought to be due to the synergistic effect of the two probes vibrating at different rates. The outer probe is approximately 1 mm shorter than the inner probe and is thought to have some ballistic effect on the stones.

In a comparative study, CyberWandTM and Lithoclast Select lithotripters had similar stone clearance rates in PCNL for stones >2 cm. The safety and efficacy of these devices were comparable [20]. However, measurement of occupational noise exposure during endourologic procedures with the CyberWandTM was noted to be significantly louder than other lithotripsy devices [21].

6.3 UreTron (Richard Wolf)

It is an electromechanical device that consists of a generator, handpiece, and probes. UreTron is a single-probe lithotripsy device with a frequency of vibration—21–22 kHz. It was approved by the Food and Drug Administration (FDA) in 2012. The handpiece is an ultrasonic transducer with piezoelectric ceramic elements. Although it is not a combined lithotripsy device, it has a new technology and merits special attention. The unique design of the UreTron system focuses more on sonic energy on the probe. It uses a unique micro-controller-based algorithm combined with an advanced physical component design, which allows this unique transmission capability to be used with flexible, semiflexible, and rigid probes. The probes had a 3.1-mm outer diameter and 2.5-mm inner diameter, although a 3.5-mm probe is available as well. The foot pedal has a hard stone and soft stone mode, each offering unique pulsing patterns meant to optimize fragmentation. Finally, fragments are sucked out. The system can aspirate stones simultaneously while operating at full power.

It has a very fast clearance stone rate (52 mm^3/min), especially for hard stones, with no differences in stone-free rates or need for secondary procedures. The malfunction rate was 16%, which is similar to that of other devices. Most of the issues were temporary and resolved. The most common issue was clogging of the device by stone debris, which was easily resolved by flushing. In addition, probe breakage can occur, which can easily be replaced by a new one [22].

6.4 ShockPulse SE™ (Olympus, Tokyo, Japan)

ShockPulse is a lithotripsy system that is the next generation of CyberWand. It was approved by the Food and Drug Administration (FDA) in 2014. This is a dual-action system for lithotripsy. It is composed of three elements: generator, shock wave transducer, and probe. The generator provides constant ultrasonic wave energy at approximately 21 kHz, along with intermittent shockwave energy at a high rate of 300 Hz. The shockwave probe has two buttons, one for high-power lithotripsy and one for standard-power lithotripsy. In addition, the handpiece transducer incorporates an adjustable suction control wheel that can rotate by approximately 20° from off to full flow.

ShockPulse technology works owing to its unique probe design. It has a return spring anteriorly for the creation of a high-energy shockwave and a back-free part that oscillates back and forth owing to vibration that sends propulsions at 300 Hz.

Probes of various sizes allow for standard percutaneous nephrolithotripsy, mini PCNL, URS lithotripsy, and bladder lithotripsy. 3.76 mm and 3.4 mm for PCNL and bladder, respectively. Mini PCNL is feasible with a 1.83 mm probe and URS lithotripsy with 1.50 and 0.95 mm probes. The latter does not allow suction. In an in vitro study, ShockPulse™ had a faster fragmentation and evacuation rate than LUS-II and Swiss LithoClast® Master [23]. The probes also had larger diameters, which could explain the faster evacuation rate [24].

6.5 Swiss Lithoclast® trilogy

The Swiss Lithoclast® Trilogy is the first device to combine an electromagnetic impactor with ultrasonic energy and suction, all in one probe. It was approved by the FDA in 2018. The trilogy consists of a pistol-grip handpiece with a disposable probe and a console used to set the treatment parameters and generate treatment energy. It can deliver ultrasonic and electromagnetic ballistic energy up to 12 Hz simultaneously or independently and has a suction function. It has a switch control pedal for both suction and energy control. Disposable probes range from 1.1 mm up to 3.9 mm (3.3–11.7 Fr). Disadvantages include the 1200 g weight of the handpiece which makes it less user friendly, leading to low physician satisfaction. It has an excellent safety profile with a downward displacement of the probe tip of 0.041 mm and a superimposed impactor-generated downward movement of 0.25 mm at 6–12 Hz [25, 26]. In vitro, the Lithoclast® Trilogy showed a superior stone clearance time compared to ShockPulse™ and Swiss Lithoclast® Select (Master) [25]. It is highly effective in both standard and mini PCNL, for which the mean stone volume clearance rates were 590.7 and 370.5 mm^3/min, respectively [26]. In a prospective nonrandomized study from ten European centers, the mean stone clearance was 65.55 mm^3/min or 945 mm^3/min calculated on 3D volume with an 83% stone-free rate on fluoroscopy screening at the end of the procedure with a 5% probe breakage [27]. In a systematic review study, Swiss Lithoclast Trilogy and ShockPulse SE were found to be equally effective, safe, and versatile for standard and mini PCNL [28]. However, newer data have shown that both lithotripsy devices do not confer any clinically meaningful advantage over older generation devices [29].

DOI: http://dx.doi.org/10.5772/intechopen.1003839

7. Conclusion

Older ballistic and ultrasonic devices are still viable with proven, time-tested efficacy, and safety over many years. New technological advances, including single-probe and dual-modality lithotripters using a combination of ultrasonic and ballistic characteristics, have excellent safety profiles. Although they were initially promising, they do not appear to be more effective than older generation devices. The advantages and disadvantages of each type of intracorporeal lithotripter must be considered when choosing a treatment modality for a given case.

Conflict of interest

The authors declare no conflict of interest.

Author details

Charalambos Kypraios, Ioannis Xoxakos, Ntiela Ntonta and Ioannis Efthimiou*
Department of Urology, General Hospital of Evaggelismos, Athens, Greece

*Address all correspondence to: efthimiou_ioannis@hotmail.com

References

[1] Mulvaney WP. Attempted disintegration of calculi by ultrasonic vibrations. The Journal of Urology. 1953;**70**(5):704-707. DOI: 10.1016/S0022-5347(17)67971-0

[2] Terhorst B, Lutzeyer W, Cichos M, Pohlman R. Die Zerstörung von Hansteinen durch Ultraschall. II. Ultraschall-Lithotriipsie von Blasensteinen [Destruction of urinary calculi by ultrasound. II. Ultrasound lithotripsy of bladder calculi]. Urology International. 1972;**27**(6):458-469. DOI: 10.1159/000279816

[3] Alken P, Hutschenreiter G, Günther R, Marberger M. Percutaneous stone manipulation. The Journal of Urology. 2017;**197**(2S):S154-S157. DOI: 10.1016/j.juro.2016.10.070

[4] Schulze H, Haupt G, Piergiovanni M, Wisard M, von Niederhausern W, Senge T. The Swiss Lithoclast: A new device for endoscopic stone disintegration. The Journal of Urology. 1993;**149**(1):15-18. DOI: 10.1016/s0022-5347(17)35985-2

[5] Hofbauer J, Höbarth K, Marberger M. Electrohydraulic versus pneumatic disintegration in the treatment of ureteral stones: A randomized, prospective trial. The Journal of Urology. 1995;**153**(3 Pt 1):623-625. DOI: 10.1097/00005392-199503000-00019

[6] Haupt G, Sabrodina N, Orlovski M, Haupt A, Krupin V, Engelmann U. Endoscopic lithotripsy with a new device combining ultrasound and lithoclast. Journal of Endourology. 2001;**15**(9):929-935. DOI: 10.1089/089277901753284161

[7] Kim SC, Matlaga BR, Tinmouth WW, Kuo RL, Evan AP, McAteer JA, et al. In vitro assessment of a novel dual probe ultrasonic intracorporeal lithotriptor. The Journal of Urology. 2007;**177**(4):1363-1365. DOI: 10.1016/j.juro.2006.11.033

[8] Terhorst B. The effect of electrohydaulic waves and ultrasound on the urothelium. Urologe A. 1975;**14**:41-45

[9] Lowe G, Knudsen BE. Ultrasonic, pneumatic and combination Intracorporeal lithotripsy for percutaneous nephrolithotomy. Journal of Endourology. 2009;**23**(10):1663-1668. DOI: 10.1089/end.2009.1533

[10] Piergiovanni M, Desgrandchamps F, Cochand-Priollet B, Janssen T, Colomer S, Teillac P, et al. Ureteral and bladder lesions after ballistic, ultrasonic, electrohydraulic, or laser lithotripsy. Journal of Endourology. 1994;**8**(4):293-299. DOI: 10.1089/end.1994.8.293

[11] Sarkissian C, Cui Y, Mohsenian K, Watts K, Gao T, Tarplin S, et al. Tissue damage from ultrasonic, pneumatic, and combination lithotripsy. Journal of Endourology. 2015;**29**(2):162-170. DOI: 10.1089/end.2014.0199

[12] Marberger M. Disintegration of renal and ureteral calculi with ultrasound. The Urologic Clinics of North America. 1983;**10**(4):729-742

[13] Noor Buchholz NP. Intracorporeal lithotripters: Selecting the optimum machine. BJU International. 2002;**89**(2):157-161. DOI: 10.1046/j.1464-4096.2001.00118.x

[14] Product catalogue. Swiss Lithoclast 2, Swiss Lithoclast Master, Swiss Lithoclast Accessories. Available from: http://med.sherl.ua/uploads/files/Product_Catalogue_Uro.pdf

[15] Keeley FX Jr, Pillai M, Smith G, Chrisofos M, Tolley DA. Electrokinetic lithotripsy: Safety, efficacy and limitations of a new form of ballistic lithotripsy. BJU International. 1999;**84**(3):261-263. DOI: 10.1046/j.1464-410x.1999.00160.x

[16] Chew BH, Arsovska O, Lange D, Wright JE, Beiko DT, Ghiculete D, et al. The Canadian StoneBreaker trial: A randomized, multicenter trial comparing the LMA StoneBreaker™ and the Swiss LithoClast® during percutaneous nephrolithotripsy. Journal of Endourology. 2011;**25**(9):1415-1419. DOI: 10.1089/end.2010.0708

[17] Wang AJ, Baldwin GT, Gabriel JC, Cocks FH, Goldsmith ZG, Iqbal MW, et al. In-vitro assessment of a new portable ballistic lithotripter with percutaneous and ureteroscopic models. Journal of Endourology. 2012;**26**(11):1500-1505. DOI: 10.1089/end.2012.0278

[18] Pietrow PK, Auge BK, Zhong P, Preminger GM. Clinical efficacy of a combination pneumatic and ultrasonic lithotrite. The Journal of Urology. 2003;**169**(4):1247-1249. DOI: 10.1097/01.ju.0000049643.18775.65

[19] Auge BK, Lallas CD, Pietrow PK, Zhong P, Preminger GM. In vitro comparison of standard ultrasound and pneumatic lithotrites with a new combination intracorporeal lithotripsy device. Urology. 2002;**60**:28-32

[20] York NE, Borofsky MS, Chew BH, Dauw CA, Paterson RF, Denstedt JD, et al. Randomized controlled trial comparing three different modalities of Lithotrites for Intracorporeal lithotripsy in percutaneous nephrolithotomy. Journal of Endourology. 2017;**31**(11):1145-1151. DOI: 10.1089/end.2017.0436

[21] Soucy F, Ko R, Denstedt JD, Razvi H. Occupational noise exposure during endourologic procedures. Journal of Endourology. Aug 2008;**22**(8):1609-1611. DOI: 10.1089/end.2008.0178

[22] Borofsky MS, El Tayeb MM, Paonessa JE, Lingeman JE. Initial experience and comparative efficacy of the UreTron: A new intracorporeal ultrasonic lithotriptor. Urology. 2015;**85**(6):1279-1283. DOI: 10.1016/j.urology.2015.03.016

[23] Chew BH, Matteliano AA, de Los RT, Lipkin ME, Paterson RF, Lange D. Benchtop and initial clinical evaluation of the ShockPulse stone eliminator in percutaneous nephrolithotomy. Journal of Endourology. 2017;**31**(2):191-197. DOI: 10.1089/end.2016.0664

[24] Axelsson TA, Cracco C, Desai M, Hasan MN, Knoll T, Montanari E, et al. Consultation on kidney stones, Copenhagen 2019: Lithotripsy in percutaneous nephrolithotomy. World Journal of Urology. 2021;**39**(6):1663-1670. DOI: 10.1007/s00345-020-03383-w

[25] Carlos EC, Wollin DA, Winship BB, Jiang R, Radvak D, Chew BH, et al. In vitro comparison of a novel single probe dual-energy lithotripter to current devices. Journal of Endourology. 2018;**32**(6):534-540. DOI: 10.1089/end.2018.0143. Epub 2018 May 11

[26] Sabnis RB, Balaji SS, Sonawane PL, Sharma R, Vijayakumar M, Singh AG, et al. EMS Lithoclast Trilogy™: An effective single-probe dual-energy lithotripter for mini and standard PCNL. World Journal of Urology. 2020;**38**(4):1043-1050. DOI: 10.1007/s00345-019-02843-2

[27] Thakare N, Tanase F, Saeb-Parsy K, Atassi N, Endriss R, Kamphuis G, et al. Efficacy and safety of the EMS Swiss

LithoClast® trilogy for PCNL: Results of the European multicentre prospective study on behalf of European section of UroTechnology. World Journal of Urology. 2021;**39**(11):4247-4253. DOI: 10.1007/s00345-021-03710-9

[28] De Stefano V, Castellani D, Somani BK, Giulioni C, Cormio A, Galosi AB, et al. Suction in percutaneous nephrolithotripsy: Evolution, development, and outcomes from experimental and clinical studies. Results from a systematic review. European Urology Focus. 2023;**S2405-4569**(23):00152-00159. DOI: 10.1016/j.euf.2023.06.010

[29] Mykoniatis I, Pyrgidis N, Tzelves L, Pietropaolo A, Juliebø-Jones P, De Coninck V, et al. Assessment of single-probe dual-energy lithotripters in percutaneous nephrolithotomy: A systematic review and meta-analysis of preclinical and clinical studies. World Journal of Urology. 2023;**41**(2):551-565. DOI: 10.1007/s00345-023-04278-2

Chapter 6

Contemporary Minimal Invasive Surgical Management of Stones in Children

Erhan Erdogan and Kemal Sarica

Abstract

Although urinary tract stone disease is less common in the pediatric age group than in adults, the increasing incidence of this problem in the last two decades, higher rate of recurrences and the difficulty of interventions make the this population very special for urologists from certain aspects. Continuity of normal renal functional status, complete stone elimination and prevention of stone recurrence are the most important parameters of treatment strategies for urologists. It has been well indicated that management and prevention of stone disease may cause serious morbidity along with a considerable financial cost. When compared with adult ones, based on the well documented metabolic derangements in approximately fifty per cent and anatomical abnormalities in approximately one third of the patients, pediatric stone formers require a detailed urological and metabolic evaluation. In order to plan the best surgical treatment, anatomical characteristics of the urinary system, the presence of obstruction and infection and the location as well as the size of the stone(s), must be taken into consideration. Anatomical and metabolic abnormalities should be treated in an effective manner on time. In addition to a vigorous medical treatment to alkalinize the urine and increase urinary citrate levels in certain cases; adequate fluid intake to increase urine volume and necessary lifestyle changes should be strongly recommended. With respect to the endourological stone management, all available alternatives can be performed in an effective and safe manner in these cases based on the technological advances, improvements in surgical instruments and most importantly experience gained from the adult population. Today, minimal (non) invasive management options for pediatric stones include extracorporeal shock wave lithotripsy (ESWL), semirigid ureteroscopy (URS), retrograde intrarenal surgery (RIRS), percutaneous nephrolithotomy (PCNL), laparoscopic, robot-assisted laparoscopic and open surgery. While URS, RIRS, PCNL, and laparoscopic procedures require more expertise, SWL is still the first most practicle, non-invasive choice for the vast majority of pediatric stones with its highly effective and safe nature resuting in higher stone-free rates. Open surgery always remains as an alternative treatment option for large and complicated stones with anatomical abnormalities.

Keywords: children, stone, management, contemporary, urolithiasis

1. Introduction

The incidence of pediatric nephrolithiasis has increased by 6–10% annually over the past 20 years [1]. Changes in lifestyle, dietary content, climate conditions along with the defined comorbidities seem to be the main factors on this aspect. Approximately 1–3% of all urinary tract stone patients treated are pediatric patients and 17% of these cases are under the age of 14. In a study, it has been reported that while the disease is more common in boys in the first 10 years of life, girls were found to be affected commonly in the second 10 years of life [2]. The incidence seems to be variable and while it is less common in developed countries such as the USA and Northern Europe, the disease has been reported to be endemic in developing countries such as India, Pakistan, Iran and Turkey, and in far eastern countries [3–5]. Considering the chemical composition of stones in the pediatric age group in developed countries, the stones are often in the form of calcium oxalate and calcium phosphate which are usually located in the upper urinary tract. In underdeveloped countries however, due to the high consumption of grain and rice as a possible etiological cause, bladder stones are more common with compositions of ammonium acid urate and uric acid.

On the other hand, published data has clearly shown that the recurrence rate of pediatric stone disease is quite high. Therefore, it is utmost important to determine the underlying metabolic as well as anatomical problems that may cause stone formation when developing rational and effective treatment strategies. Anatomical abnormal conditions such as ureteropelvic junction stenosis, megaureter, ureteral cyst and urethral valve are the main causes of stasis and stone formation in these cases. Concerning the metabolic aspect of the disease, hypercalciuria, hypocitraturia, hyperoxaluria, hyperuricaciduria, cystinuria and hypomagnesuria are the most commonly identified risk factors causing stone formation in children. Last but not least, endemic factors and recurrent urinary tract infections are the other most important underlying causes to be considered [6, 7].

2. Minimal invasive surgical management

Pediatric urinary tract stone disease is prone to recurrence, so all necessary precautions should be taken to reduce the recurrences. Additionally, minimal invasive surgical options need to be performed tor ender these cases stone free reduce the possible negative effects of surgery on the growing kidneys. Surgical treatment is recommended for ureteral stones unlikely for spontaneous passage and that of symptomatic kidney stones [8]. Surgical treatment of pediatric stone patients has become more effective and safe with the development of miniature endourological devices in parallel with technological developments and the increase in the endourological surgical experience of urologists. The same minimally invasive surgical methods are used in pediatric patients as in the adult population. Commonly used minimally invasive methods are ureteroscopy (URS), shock wave lithotripsy (SWL) and percutaneous nephrolithotomy (PCNL). Although patients are at risk of anesthesia and radiation during the application of these methods, they are considered minimally invasive compared to more invasive surgeries such as open or laparoscopic surgery performed in patients with anatomical anomalies.

As in adults, the aim of treatment in pediatric patients is to achieve the highest SFR without the least number of procedures and complications. The equipment, localization and size of the stone(s), anatomical factors, comorbidities and the experience of the surgeon must be taken into consideration when choosing the type of the procedure.

There is still no consensus on the definition of stone-free status after these procedures an Tasian et al. defined stone-free as "resolution of symptoms by clearance of the offending stone on imaging after ureteroscopy, shock wave lithotripsy, percutaneous nephrolithotomy or spontaneous stone passage" [9]. However, in clinical practice, there is no established consensus on the size stone fragments give clinical symptoms and spontaneous passage in pediatric patients [10].

3. Extracorporeal shock wave lithotripsy (ESWL)

The minimally invasive ESWL method works on the principle of high-energy shock waves generated from the electrodes in the lithotripsy device. There are three types of shock wave generators. Electrohydraulic generators use evaporation bubbles, electromagnetic generators use magnetic fields and piezoelectric generators work on the principle of vibration of crystals when current flows through them [10, 11]. This method, which allows kidney stones to be broken into small pieces that will allow spontaneous passage, was introduced into clinical use in the 1980s and has proven its effectiveness and reliability over time. Since it is minimally invasive and effective, it has become the first choice for stone treatment in pediatric patients. Initially, its use in pediatric patients was delayed due to concerns about adverse consequences that may develop after administration due to organ development in children [12]. Over time, these concerns disappeared, and SWL began to be widely used in pediatric stone patients. SWL has been the first choice in the treatment of pediatric stone diseases because of the positive effects such as less stone-skin distance and better dilatation of the ureters allowing shorter and spontaneous stone passage in children [13].

SWL has more effective aspects in children than adults. In children, shock wave energy attenuation is less due to the short stone-skin distance. In addition, since the water content of the tissues between the body surface and the kidney tissue in children is higher than in adults, the acoustic impedance is low, which is very convenient for the transmission of energy.

The undesirable aspect of SWL is that several sessions may be required and some patients may need additional interventions to ensure stone-free status. Contraindications for its application are coagulation dysfunction, active urinary tract infection, extreme obesity, skeletal malformations and hemangioma located close to the stone. In the light of the literature data, the SFR seems to be high in renal pelvis and calyx stones up to 2 cm. However, as the stone size increases, lower success rates could be anticipated in cases with calcium oxalate monohydrate and cystine stones or in difficult access situations due to the anomalies of urinary tract [14].

Approximately 80% of stones seen in pediatric patients can successfully be treated with SWL. While short-term stone-free rates are 57–97%, there are different studies reporting that this rate is 57–92% in the long-term [15–17].

Because of the relative hardness of cystine stones and their resistance to high energy shock waves, SWL is not considered as the first choice in the treatment of these calculi [18]. As mentioned above, kids with a history of anatomical abnormalities are not ideal candidates for SWL because stone-free rates are as low as 12.5% in such patients [19]. Although general anesthesia is usually performed in young children, in older children sedation could be sufficient to relieve possible discomfort during the SWL procedure [20, 21].

Hematuria resulting from local trauma caused by the application shock waves is the most common complication after SWL. Haematuria usually resolves spontaneously within 1 week [22, 23]. In addition, renal colic, steinstrasse, subcapsular haematoma, perirenal haematoma, intestinal perforation, hepatic haematoma, splenic rupture, abdominal aortic rupture, pneumothorax, urinothorax and acute necrotising pancreatitis are possible complications of SWL [14]. Care should also be taken in terms of the potential risk of hypertension. A population-based retrospective study found that SWL for the kidney stones was associated with a 40% higher risk of hypertension, and patients treated with SWL had twice the risk of hypertension than those without kidney stones [24, 25]. Similar data is highly limited in children but the potential risk of hypertension should always be taken into account given the long life expectancy. Although potential hypertension and loss of renal function have been seriously discussed, no significant morphological and functional changes were detected in long-term evaluations of children treated in different series. However, it should not be forgotten that pediatric patients should be completely stone free in a short time with a reasonable number (up to 2000) of high energy shock waves [26, 27].

Ureteral stones sizing less than 5 mm tend to pass spontaneously at a rate of 98%. Very successful results are obtained with SWL in the treatment of impacted ureteral stones larger than 5 mm [11, 20, 28]. Compared with adults in terms of anatomy and elasticity of the ureter, pediatric patients pass stone fragments more easily and ureteral stent placement is rarely needed. Alternative surgical procedures such as PNL or RIRS should be considered in cases where the stone size is large and a ureteral stent may be needed.

In conclusion, available evidence-based data suggest that SWL is an effective and safe treatment alternative in the majority of pediatric stones.

4. Ureteroscopy (URS)

As an highly effective and safe management option, URS, has been easily adopted and applied in adult patients. However, it took a reasonable time period to be applied in children due to the lack of experience, the small size of the body and concerns about intraoperative complications. URS was first applied to distal ureteral stones in children in 1988, and a stone-free rates of 86–100% has been reported [29]. Parallel to technological developments, with the introduction of thinner and more flexible ureteroscopic instruments and efficient use of Holmium: YAG laser, this procedure has begun to be used and preferred not only in distal and middle ureteral stones but also in the upper ureteral ones. Literature data showing similar or even better results than adult case applications in terms of treatment efficacy and complication rates of URS [30, 31]. Concerns about damage to the ureteral and urethral mucosa related to the use of thick-calibrated (11.5 Fr-8.5 Fr) instruments have disappeared with the clinical introduction of thinner (4.5/6 Fr, 6/7.5 Fr and 8/9.8 Fr) caliber instruments. Therefore, currently complications arising from the use of larger instruments are very rare. There are two types of ureteroscopic instruments in different calibers for the removal of ureterla and kidney stones namely, semi-rigid and flexible. When these two models are compared, the semi-rigid model appears to have a larger working channel, better water flow and greater durability. With the cautious use of semi-rigid model, the entire ureter and even the pelvic system (in a very careful approach in limited cases) can be accessed. The flexible model is more suitable for upper ureteral stones particular in kinked ureters due to its bendable tip [32].

SWL or URS is recommended for pediatric upper urinary tract stones which do not pass with follow-up or medical expulsive therapy, or who have a very low probability of spontaneous passage. Published data on this aspect demonstrated that, the SFR is 78% for stones >10 mm and 95% for stones <10 mm when treated with URS. Compared to SWL, this rate is 73 and 87%, respectively [8].

URS treatment of upper ureteral stones requires advanced endoscopic skills and the risk of ureteral trauma is very high, especially during the removal of large and impacted stones. For lower and middle ureteral stones, stone-free rates are satisfactory ranging between 87.5 and 100% in different studies [11, 31].

In recent years, URS has also gained popularity in the management of pediatric ureteral stones and has become widely used for stones <15 mm. It should be kept in mind that the procedure is not complication free despite the surgical experience gained and widespread use of the fine and less traumatic instruments. In general, complication rates in children are similar to the rates noted in adults [33]. Potential complications include ureteral avulsion, ureteral perforation, hematuria, infection, and ureteral stricture. If ureteral perforation occurs, the procedure should be terminated and a ureteral stent placed. If a ureteral avulsion occurs, which is a very rare but very serious complication, extensive, judicious approaches including open repair will be required. In a study, the complication rate of URS in children was reported as 7.1% [34]. There are certain concerns about the role and necessity of ureteral dilatation and complications such as urethral stricture and vesicoureteral reflux may occur after this maneuver. However, studies have shown that such risks have not been increased [35].

5. Retrograde intrarenal surgery (RIRS)

Similar to adult patients, the main goal of the treatment for pediatric kidney stones is to achieve a stone-free kidney with the least number of interventions resulting in the least morbidity. As a result of the marked developments in the ureteral access sheat, guide wire, nitinol basket and holmium laser fiber technology used in endoscopic surgery the application rates of RIRS in pediatric stone patients has also increased. Recent data have shown that RIRS can be performed also in pediatric renal stones larger than 2 cm [36]. At the same time, the use of natural orifice approach to reach the stone and the high success with low morbidity increased the popularity of RIRS. This makes RIRS more effective and safe in the treatment of pediatric kidney Stones when compared with PNL.

Currently the EAU guidelines recommended RIRS as another treatment method in addition to SWL and PCNL for the minimal invasive and relatively safe treatment of kidney stones [37]. Initially, the indications for RIRS were limited to lower calyx stones, stones smaller than 1.5 cm and Stones resistant to SWL. However, these limitations in RIRS indications have decreased due to the recent accumulated experience and the ease of application provided by the advances in surgical instruments. RIRS is an acceptable treatment option in kids where SWL was found to be unsuccessful for pediatric kidney stones smaller than 2 cm. Because of its relatively low morbidity in pediatric kidney stones larger than 2 cm, it is also an alternative treatment option to PCNL in experienced hands. Li et al. treated 55 pediatric patients with upper ureteral and kidney stones with RIRS and reported a stone-free rate of 94% [38]. In a study Resorlu et al., have compared 106 patients with kidney stones undergoing mini-PCNL and 95 patients undergoing RIRS based on the SFR obtained and reported outcomes were 86 and 84%, respectively [39]. Despite similar SFR, RIRS appears to be safer because of less radiation exposure, fewer complications, instrumental administration through the natural orifice urinary tract which minimizes well the extent of possible trauma to tissues.

RIRS can be applied effectively and safely also in certain problematic cases such as the ones with non-opaque stones, SWL resistant stones, anatomical abnormalities, lower calyceal calculi, musculoskeletal deformities as well as obesity.

In summary based on the safe applications and successful outcomes in experienced hands, RIRS could be regarded as an effective and safe method in the treatment of pediatric kidney stones. However, it should be kept in mind that that uncorrected bleeding disorder, uncontrolled urinary tract infection, severe urethral stricture, narrow ureter, large and complex stones, anatomical abnormalities that make retrograde access difficult and previous endoscopic failures are absolute contraindications for this particular procedure.

6. Percutaneous nephrolithotomy (PCNL)

PCNL in pediatric kidney stone treatment was first performed in 1985 [40]. The EUA guidelines for stones recommend PCNL for the treatment of complex (staghorn or partially staghorn), kidney stones larger than 2 cm, lower calyx stones larger than 1 cm, kidney and ureteral stones that have failed SWL and RIRS [14]. Although PNL has been widely used in adult patients, it took a certain time period to become widespread in pediatric patients due to concerns regarding the indications and large sized instruments used at first. However, the miniaturization of the tools used as a result of technological advances paved the way for widespread use of PNL in children. In their original study Jackman et al. emphasized that the 24 Fr sheath used in pediatric patients is actually equivalent to the use of a 72 Fr sheath in adults [41] which certainly justifies the initial concerns discussed above. Taking the certain level of damage induced in the kidney parenchyma, miniaturization of instruments has resulted in the limitation of severe complication such as bleeding and shortened the operative times.

The patient's age and stone volume are very important factors in selection of appropriate instruments. Although definitions vary according to the size of the instruments used, they are generally defined as mini (16/22 Fr), super-mini (14/16 Fr), ultra-mini (10/13 Fr) and micro (4.85 Fr). This miniaturization of the instruments has enabled them to be used in pediatric patients of all age groups. This has made PCNL an alternative as an option in the treatment of smaller stones that are candidates for SWL or RIRS. It also increases tubeless PCNL experiences, resulting in reduced pain and reduced hospital stays. Decreased calibration of instruments brings with it limitations such as reduced image quality, difficulty in removing stone fragments and higher intrarenal pressure. However, the introduction of vacuum-assisted evacuation sheaths can help solve these problems and shorten operation times [42].

Mini-PCNL is a modified PCNL procedure using a smaller (14–20 Fr) channel. Zeng et al. treated 20 children with kidney stones with mini-PCNL and reported a SFR of 95% [43]. Mini-PCNL has advantages such as reduction in bleeding, postoperative pain and hospital stay, and reduction in treatment costs.

Zeng et al. designed a new miniaturized endoscopic system called super-mini PCNL (SMP) to further optimize the PCNL technique. It was designed with a two-layer metal structure with 12 or 14 Fr nephroscope options associated with a new irrigation suction sheath concept [44]. This new design can prevent the possible rise in intrarenal pressure, improve image quality and improve stone fragment removal by continuous aspiration of the dust and fragments as they form during the procedure.

Desai et al. proposed a new PCNL procedure, which they called ultra-mini PCNL. The aim here was to increase the efficacy and safety of mini-PCNL and to reduce complications. In this definition, 11 or 13 Fr sheath, 7.5 Fr nephroscope and 3 Fr telescope are used [45]. There are indications for the use of this modality as an alternative to SWL or RIRS in SWL-resistant stones, renal diverticulum stones, lower calyx stones that are not suitable for RIRS or medium-sized kidney stones. Dede et al. reported a stone-free rate of 87.1% for kidney stones managed with ultra-mini PCNL. They reported that no patient required blood transfusion and the safety of the operation was increased due to the low intrarenal pressure during the procedure [46].

Last but last least, another version of mini-PCNL was described as micro-PCNL by Desai et al. With the help of 4.8 Fr tract size, the procedure is performed in a single step with the careful use of an "all-seeing" needle [47]. This system has been advised to be performed in both pediatric and adult patients with relatively smaller (1–2 cm) stones. This modality seems to have some advantages such as no tract dilatation, less bleeding, less exposure to radiation, shorter operation time and less complications. However, the modality has been found to have certain disadvantages where the quality of vision was found to be not clear enough and expensive nature of the applications. Patients regarded to be unsuitable for SWL due to anatomical abnormalities may be a good indication for micro-PCNL.

7. Laparoscopic surgery

Laparoscopic procedures can be used in the treatment of pediatric renal and ureteral calculi, but since the data reported in the literature are very limited, large series are needed. Therefore, laparoscopic and robot-assisted pyelolithotomy, nephrolithotomy or ureterolithotomy may be an option only in selected patients with large renal pelvic and ureteral calculi. The EAU stone guidelines suggests that laparoscopic or robot-assisted intervention may be considered for complicated renal anatomy, calyceal diverticulum, megaureter or after a failed endoscopic intervention [14].

8. Cystolithotomy

Bladder stones, which are reported to be an endemic pathology in underdeveloped and developing countries, are also seen after augmented bladder or continent urinary diversion. The treatment principles of bladder stones are like upper urinary tract stones. Alternative methods such as transurethral, percutaneous suprapubic lithotripsy or suprapubic cystolithotomy are available in the treatment of bladder stones, which are generally seen as single and hard chemical structures. The biggest drawback of transurethral treatment options is the damage that may occur, especially in the male urethra [48].

9. Conclusions

The main goal of pediatric kidney stone management is to protect the renal function as much as possible, achieve the highest SFR in a single session (if possible) and prevent further recurrences. While planning the most rational treatment option, stone and the patient related factors need to be very well evaluated. The individual experience of the surgeon is also another highly important parameter that should be taken into account for successful and complication free outcomes particularly in this specific population.

Although data showing that SWL and URS are equally effective and safe alternatives in the minimal invasive treatment of stones sizing 1–2 cm, similar to the clinical applications in adult patients, SWL is still considered to be the first treatment option for such kidney stones. PCNL remains the most effective method for the treatment of large and complicated pediatric kidney Stones sizing larger than 2 cm. Further data indicating the exact role of laparoscopic and robot-assisted pyelolithotomy and even RIRS methods are certainly needed.

Well-designed, randomized studies are still needed to understand better the exact role and judicious use of RIRS and that of different miniaturized PCNL methods.

Funding support

None.

Conflicts of interest

The authors declare no conflict of interest.

Author details

Erhan Erdogan[1*] and Kemal Sarica[1,2]

1 Department of Urology, Health Sciences University, Sancaktepe Sehit Prof. Dr. Ilhan Varank Research and Training Hospital, Istanbul, Turkey

2 Department of Urology, Medical School, Biruni University, Istanbul, Turkey

*Address all correspondence to: erhandr@hotmail.com

References

[1] Van Batavia JP, Tasian GE. Clinical effectiveness in the diagnosis and acute management of pediatric nephrolithiasis. International Journal of Surgery (London, England). 2016;**36**:698-704

[2] Dwyer ME, Krambeck AE, Bergstralh EJ, Milliner DS, Lieske JC, Rule AD. Temporal trends in incidence of kidney stones among children: A 25-year population based study. The Journal of Urology. 2012;**188**:247-252

[3] Sarica K. Pediatric urolithiasis: Etiology, specific pathogenesis and medical treatment. Urological Research. 2006;**24**:1-6

[4] Kroovand RL. Pediatrik ürolitiazis. Urologic Clinics of North America. 1997;**12**:173-177

[5] Sepahi MA, Heidari A, Shajari A. Clinical manifestations and etiology of renal stones in children less than 14 years age. Saudi Journal of Kidney Diseases and Transplantation. 2010;**21**:181-184

[6] Nicoletta JA, Lande MB. Medical evaluation and treatment of urolithiasis. Pediatric Clinics of North America. 2006;**53**:479-491

[7] Sarica K, Erturhan S, Yurtseven C, Yagci F. Effect of potassium citrate therapy on stone recurrence and regrowth after extracorporeal shockwave lithotripsy in children. Journal of Endourology. 2006;**20**:875-879

[8] Assimos D, Krambeck A, Miller NL, Monga M, Murad MH, Nelson CP, et al. Surgical management of stones. American Urological Association/ Endourological Society Guideline, Part I. The Journal of Urology. 2016;**196**:1153-1160

[9] Tasian GE, Kabarriti AE, Kalmus A, Furth SL. Kidney stone recurrence among children and adolescents. The Journal of Urology. 2017;**197**:246-252

[10] Manzoor H, Saikali WS. Renal Extracorporeal Lithotripsy. Treasure Island, FL, USA: StatPearls; 2022

[11] Lahme S. Shockwave lithotripsy and endourological stone treatment in children. Urological Research. 2006;**34**:112-117

[12] Lifshitz DA, Lingeman JE, Zafar FS, Hollensbe DW, Nyhuis AW, Evan AP. Alterations in predicted growth rates of pediatric kidneys treated with extracorporeal shockwave lithotripsy. Journal of Endourology. 1998;**12**:469-475

[13] McAdams S, Shukla AR. Pediatric extracorporeal shock wave lithotripsy: Predicting successful outcomes. Indian Journal of Urology. 2010;**26**:544-548

[14] ESWL in children: EAU Guidelines. In: Proceedings of the EAU Annual Congress Amsterdam, Amsterdam, The Netherlands, 1-4 July 2022. Arnhem, The Netherlands: EAU Guidelines Office; 2022

[15] Schultz-Lampel D, Lampel A. The surgical management of stones in children. BJU International. 2001;**87**:732-740

[16] Rizvi S, Nagvi S, Hussain Z, et al. Management of pediatric urolithiasis in Pakistan. Experience with 1440 children. The Journal of Urology. 2003;**169**:634-638

[17] Landau E, Gofrit O, Shapiro A, et al. Extracorporeal shockwave lithotripsy is highly effective for ureteral calculi

in children. Journal of Urology. 2001;**165**:2316-2318

[18] Landau EH, Shenfeld OZ, Pode D, Shapiro A, Meretyk S, Katz G, et al. Extracorporeal shock wave lithotripsy in prepubertal children: 22-year experience at a single institution with a single lithotriptor. The Journal of Urology. 2009;**182**:1835-1839

[19] Nelson CP, Diamond DA, Cendron M, Peters CA, Cilento BG. Extracorporeal shock wave lithotripsy in pediatric patients using a late generation portable lithotriptor: Experience at Children's Hospital Boston. The Journal of Urology. 2008;**180**:1865-1868

[20] Cass AS. Comparison of First-Generation (Dornier HM3) and Second Generation (Medstone STS) Lithotriptors: Treatment results with 145 renal and ureteral calculi in children. Journal of Endourology. 1996;**10**:493

[21] Egilmez T, Tekin MI, Gonen M, Kilinc F, Goren R, Ozkardes H. Efficacy and safety of a new-generation shockwave lithotripsy machine in the treatment of single renal or ureteral stones: Experience with 2670 patients. Journal of Endourology. 2007;**21**:23-27

[22] Yucel S, Akin Y, Danisman A, Guntekin E. Complications and associated factors of pediatric extracorporeal shock wave lithotripsy. The Journal of Urology. 2012;**187**:1812-1816

[23] Akin Y, Yucel S. Long-term effects of pediatric extracorporeal shockwave lithotripsy on renal function. Research and Reports in Urology. 2014;**6**:21-25

[24] Denburg MR, Jemielita TO, Tasian GE, Haynes K, Mucksavage P, Shults J, et al. Assessing the risk of incident hypertension and chronic kidney disease after exposure to shock wave lithotripsy and ureteroscopy. Kidney International. 2016;**89**:185-192

[25] Shang W, Li Y, Ren Y, Yang Y, Li H, Dong J. Nephrolithiasis and risk of hypertension: A meta-analysis of observational studies. BMC Nephrology. 2017;**18**:344

[26] Frick J, Sarica K, Kohle R, et al. Long-term follow-up after to extracorporeal shock wave lithotripsy in children. European Urology. 1991;**19**:225-229

[27] Brinkmann O, Griehl A, Kuwertz-Broking E, et al. Extracorporeal shock wave lithotripsy in children. European Urology. 2001;**39**:591-594

[28] Demirkesen O, Tansu N, Yaycioglu O. Extracorporeal shockwave lithotripsy in the pediatric population. Journal of Endourology. 1999;**13**:147-150

[29] Ritchey M, Patterson DE, Kelalis PP, Segura JW. A case of pediatric ureteroscopic lasertripsy. The Journal of Urology. 1988;**139**:1272-1274

[30] Bassiri A, Ahmadnia H, Darabi MR, Yonessi M. Transureteral lithotripsy in pediatric practice. Journal of Endourology. 2002;**16**:257-260

[31] Zheng W, Denstedt JD. Intracorporeal lithotripsy. The Urologic Clinics of North America. 2000;**27**:301-313

[32] Citamak B, Mammadov E, Kahraman O, Ceylan T, Dogan HS, Tekgul S. Semi-rigid ureteroscopy should not be the first option for proximal ureteral stones in children. Journal of Endourology. 2018;**32**:1028-1032

[33] Minevich E, Defoor W, Reddy P, Nishinaka K, Wacksman J, Sheldon C, et al. Ureteroscopy is safe and effective in prepubertal children. The Journal of Urology. 2005;**174**:276-279

[34] Ishii H, Griffin S, Somani BK. Ureteroscopy for stone disease in the paediatric population: A systematic review. BJU International. 2015;**115**:867-873

[35] Al Busaidy SS, Prem AR, Mehdat M. Pediatric ureteroscopy for ureteric calculi: A 4-year experience. British Journal of Urology. 1997;**80**:797-801

[36] Akman T, Binbay M, Ozgor F, Ugurlu M, Tekinarslan E, Kezer C, et al. Comparison of percutaneous nephrolithotomy and retrograde flexible nephrolithotripsy for the management of 2-4 cm stones: A matched-pair analysis. BJU International. 2012;**109**:1384-1389

[37] Türk C, Petrik A, Sarica K, Seitz C, Skolarikos A, Straub M, et al. EAU guidelines on interventional treatment of urolithiasis. European Urology. 2016;**69**:475-482

[38] Li J, Xiao J, Han T, Tian Y, Wang W, Du Y. Flexible ureteroscopic lithotripsy for the treatment of upper urinary tract calculi in infants. Experimental Biology and Medicine (Maywood, N.J.). 2017;**242**:153-159

[39] Resorlu B, Oguz U, Resorlu EB, Oztuna D, Unsal A. The impact of pelvicaliceal anatomy on the success of retrograde intrarenal surgery in patients with lower pole renal stones. Urology. 2012;**79**:61-66. DOI: 10.1016/j.urology.2011.06.031

[40] Woodside JR, Stevens GF, Stark GL, Borden TA, Ball WS. Percutaneous stone removal in children. The Journal of Urology. 1985;**134**:1166-1167. DOI: 10.1016/S0022-5347(17)47669-5

[41] Jackman SV, Hedican SP, Peters CA, et al. Percutaneous nephrolithotomy in infants and preschool children: Experience with a new technique. Urology. 1998;**52**:697-701

[42] Zanetti SP, Lievore E, Fontana M, et al. Vacuum-assisted mini-percutaneous nephrolithotomy: A new perspective in fragments clearance and intrarenal pressure control. World Journal of Urology. 2021;**39**:1717-1723

[43] Zeng G, Zhao Z, Zhao Z, Yuan J, Wu W, Zhong W. Percutaneous nephrolithotomy in infants: Evaluation of a single-center experience. Urology. 2012;**80**:408-411. DOI: 10.1016/j.urology.2012.04.058

[44] Zeng G, Wan S, Zhao Z, Zhu J, Tuerxun A, Song C, et al. Super-mini percutaneous nephrolithotomy (SMP): A new concept in technique and instrumentation. BJU International. 2016;**117**:655-661

[45] Desai J, Zeng G, Zhao Z, Zhong W, Chen W, Wu W, et al. Novel technique of ultra-mini-percutaneous nephrolithotomy: Introduction and an initial experience for treatment of upper urinary calculi less than 2 cm. BioMed Research International. 2013;**2013**:490793

[46] Dede O, Sancaktutar AA, Dagguli M, Utangac M, Bas O, Penbegul N. Ultra-mini-percutaneous nephrolithotomy in pediatric nephrolithiasis: Both low pressure and high efficiency. Journal of Pediatric Urology. 2015;**11**(253):e1-e6

[47] Desai MR, Sharma R, Mishra S, Sabnis RB, Stief C, Bader M. Single-step percutaneous nephrolithotomy (microperc): The initial clinical report. The Journal of Urology. 2011;**186**:140-145

[48] Papatsoris AG, Varkarakis I, Dellis A, Deliveliotis C. Bladder lithiasis: From open surgery to lithotripsy. Urological Research. 2006;**34**:163-167